2-6-12

W9-BMP-072

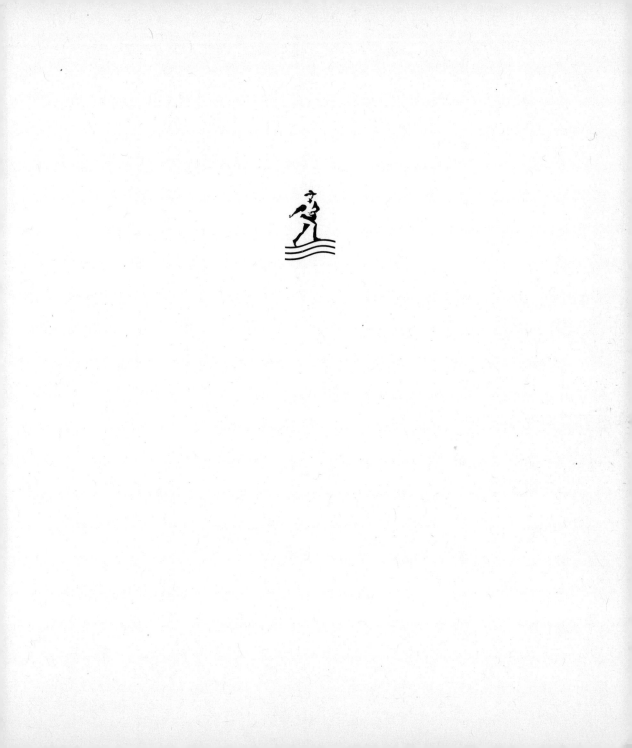

ALSO BY BOB GREENE

The Best Life Guide to Managing Diabetes and Pre-Diabetes

The Best Life Diet Cookbook

The Best Life Diet

The Best Life Diet Daily Journal

Bob Greene's Total Body Makeover

The Get with the Program! Guide to Good Eating

Get with the Program!

Keep the Connection: Choices for a Better Body and a Healthier Life

Make the Connection: Ten Steps to a Better Body—and a Better Life

BOB GREENE

ANN KEARNEY-COOKE, PhD
JANIS JIBRIN, MS, RD

THE LIFE YOU WANT

GET MOTIVATED, LOSE WEIGHT, AND BE HAPPY

SIMON & SCHUSTER

NEW YORK   LONDON   TORONTO   SYDNEY

Simon & Schuster
1230 Avenue of the Americas
New York, NY 10020

First Simon & Schuster hardcover edition January 2011

SIMON & SCHUSTER and colophon are registered trademarks of Simon & Schuster, Inc.

For information about special discounts for bulk purchases, please contact Simon & Schuster
Special Sales at 1-866-506-1949 or business@simonandschuster.com.

The Simon & Schuster Speakers Bureau can bring authors to your live event. For more information
or to book an event contact the Simon & Schuster Speakers Bureau at 1-866-248-3049 or visit our
website at www.simonspeakers.com.

Manufactured in the United States of America

1   3   5   7   9   10   8   6   4   2

Library of Congress Cataloging-in-Publication Data

Greene, Bob (Bob W.)
The life you want: Get motivated, lose weight, and be happy / Bob Greene,
Ann Kearney-Cooke, and Janis Jibrin.
p.   cm.
Includes bibliographical references and index.
1. Weight loss—Psychological aspects. I. Kearney-Cooke, Ann Mary
II. Jibrin, Janis. III. Title.
RM222.2.G7227 2011
613.2'5—dc22
2010027534

ISBN 978-1-4165-8836-8
ISBN 978-1-4391-9006-7 (ebook)

ACKNOWLEDGMENTS

With special thanks to Donna Fennessy and Daryn Eller for their outstanding contributions to this book. And to Dianne Tieger for her research help, and Beth McGilley, PhD, for her thoughtful comments on the manuscript. We're also very grateful to those who shared their weight-loss success stories, as well as to all the other clients, patients, readers of our books, and members of *TheBestLife.com* whose perseverance and courage to make tough changes in their lives are a constant source of inspiration. We were very fortunate to gather insights from the accomplished researchers who provided essential background information, including Eric Stice, PhD, and Ronald Krauss, MD, as well as those who were quoted throughout the book: Adrian Brown, MD, Stephanie Fulton, PhD, Michael J. Joyner, MD, Marcia Pelchat, PhD, Suzanne Phelan, PhD, Angela Taylor, LCSW, Pedro J. Teixeira, PhD, Inga Treitler, PhD, and Paul K. Whelton, MB, MD, MSC.

CONTENTS

INTRODUCTION

By Bob Greene

SOME OF THE MOST vivid memories of my childhood are the trips I used to take with my family to visit my grandmother and great-grandmother. The two of them lived together a short distance from our suburban home, and every few weeks or so, my parents would pack us kids into the car and hit the turnpike to make the twenty-five-minute drive to Camden, New Jersey. I'd hear my mom calling for me—I was inevitably outside riding my bike, kicking a ball around, or playing catch with a friend—and I'd hop into the backseat, reluctant to stop what I was doing but always happy to see my grandmother and great-grandmother once we reached our destination.

What was unusual about the experience, though, was that my great-grandmother was bedridden. I can't remember ever seeing her get out of bed. And of course she was never able to come outside and play with my sister and me. Instead we would talk to her while standing on top of a chair that had been placed next to her bed for visitors.

The "party line" on my great-grandmother was that she was immobile because of a bad knee. When I was older, it occurred to me that the knee story was just a nice way of saying that she was too overweight to get around. But back then nobody referred to her weight problem, and if my great-grandmother was at all bothered by the state she was in, she kept it well hidden from us kids. Since I was so young, I accepted her situation just the way it was, but I think that deep down I also sensed that her days could have been better. My world was all about running, jumping, kicking, climbing—I was always moving—so even at a young age, I was aware that someone who is bedridden misses out on many of the joys of life. That isn't to say that there weren't good times. Those visits with my great-grandmother were fun, and she always seemed to have a great outlook. But as I reflect on it now, it's sad that her life was so limited—especially because it didn't have to be that way.

I often think about my great-grandmother when I work with clients, write about weight loss, or simply when I hear some statistic about the dismal rate of weight loss success in this country. Only a small percentage of people who lose a significant amount of weight end up keeping it off, and the burning question, of course, is *Why?* Why do most people who change their eating and exercise habits change them right back again? What is it that prevents them from pursuing better health and a life of greater physical ease? And what is so special about the people who do succeed at long-term weight loss? What are they doing that the majority of Americans aren't?

I'll never know exactly what prevented my great-grandmother from losing enough weight to get back on her feet again, but she must have been facing issues far deeper than just the challenge of reining in her eating. At the time, without the insight I would gain years later while working with people struggling to slim down, it just seemed like a sad yet unpreventable situation. Nevertheless, I was curious—and still am—about why my great-grandmother had to live such a restricted life.

I know that most kids would have just shrugged off the fact that an older relative was bedridden. However—and sometimes to the annoyance of my parents—I was never like most kids when it came to matters of health and well-being. I can barely remember a time when I wasn't conscious of what was good for you and what was bad for you, and that was particularly true when it came to my family's diet. Like most families at the time, we were meat and potatoes eaters, although we also always had a variety of vegetables on our dinner plates. My mom was somewhat ahead of her time in that respect, always serving vegetables of different colors—say, green spinach and yellow squash—to give us an assortment of vitamins.

So, overall, our diet wasn't bad—only, I wanted it to be better. Anytime my parents would serve foods that I'd heard were unhealthy, I'd be quick to call them on it. I'd read a newspaper article about how nitrates were linked to cancer, and I'd refuse bacon with breakfast. Salt? It causes high blood pressure, Mom! Long before the fat-free revolution of the eighties and nineties, I was trimming the fat off my meat at the dinner table and urging everyone else to do the same. To my parents, I was just Bob being Bob—a little odd, but they loved me anyway.

Perhaps I was a bit over the top, but it's also true that my family had genuine health concerns. Many of my relatives, not just my great-grandmother, battled with their weight, and my dad was a smoker. To his credit, he eventually quit, but when I was a teenager, he was still going at it, and it really bothered me. One time my family planned to take a great cross-country road trip in an RV, and I opted to stay home. I told my parents it was because someone had to take care of the dogs, but the truth was that I didn't want to spend weeks trapped in a cabin on wheels cloudy with my dad's cigarette smoke.

This early interest in health and fitness seemed to foretell my future—and, of course, I would eventually seek a career in that direction. But it wasn't a straight line from counseling my parents at the dinner table to counseling clients. There were many other subjects I was passionate about, too, some of which I considered pursuing as a profession. Among them was a somewhat precocious fascination with psychology. One of the books I discovered and, oddly, enjoyed reading at the tender age of about thirteen was Abraham Maslow's *Toward a Psychology of Being*. I still have my old yellowing, highlighted copy. Maslow, known as the father of humanistic psychology, classified the motives that drive human beings into five levels and shaped them into a pyramid called the hierarchy of needs. At the bottom of the pyramid are basic needs like those for food and water. According to Maslow, it is only when we satisfy those needs that we will be motivated to move up to higher levels and seek things such as love and self-esteem. At the top of his pyramid is self-actualization: the need to reach your potential as a person. Maslow's take on human nature revealed a deep understanding of the human psyche, and I continue to be influenced by it today.

When it came time for me to go to college, I was offered a soccer scholarship to Brandeis University in Boston, where Maslow had been chairman of the psychology department for two decades before he died in 1970. I gave serious consideration to attending the school and studying psychology. However, I was also drawn in a different direction, and, in the end, I turned down the scholarship and opted to go to the University of Delaware, where I studied health and physical education. I would later earn a graduate degree from the University of Arizona in exercise physiology, emphasizing metabolism and weight loss. But my fascination with the way the mind works also endured, and I took psychology courses all through college and kept reading psychology books on my own.

Psychology was mostly a personal interest; I didn't expect that it would have much to do with my chosen career as an exercise physiologist specializing in fitness and weight loss. But the more I worked with clients struggling to change their eating and exercise habits, the clearer it became to me that psychology has *everything* to do with fitness and weight loss. While it's important to have good diet and exercise strategies in place, I've never met anyone who was able to stick with healthy eating and physical activity if he didn't have his emotional and psychological life in order. Going back to some of the questions I mentioned earlier—Why do most people who change their eating and exercise habits change them right back again? What is it that prevents them from pursuing better health and a life of greater physical ease?—I think I can say with some certainty that, contrary to what people often think, the biggest barriers to long-term weight loss aren't ineffective diets or inadequate exercise plans.

In most cases, the biggest barriers to losing weight and keeping it off are related to the way you think, how you feel, and how you manage your life.

Early on in my career, I began working with clients who'd tell me that although they initially had no problem following a nutritious eating plan and ramping up their physical activity, they'd let their new habits slide after a while. When I'd ask, "Why did you give that up?" rarely did anyone have a viable answer. So I'd probe more. "How was your life when you were eating right and exercising?" Inevitably, they'd always say, "My life was great!" Never did I hear "My life was terrible when I was eating right, exercising, and taking care of myself." As I got to know them better, I would usually learn that body weight wasn't the only issue they were trying to manage. In most cases, they were also dealing with—or *not* dealing with—some kind of deeply rooted emotional or psychological issue, or they were simply having trouble managing their lives.

When you try to lose weight without tackling the underlying issues that cause you to overeat and choose a sedentary life in the first place, the odds against your success are significant. And the underlying issues I'm talking about can take many forms. Maybe you're in the grip of a bad relationship; it's hard to make healthful changes when you don't have the support of a significant other or if the drama of that relationship drives you to take comfort in food. Maybe your efforts to cope with the stress of financial troubles, overwork, or a bad job are sucking up the energy you need to lead a healthier life. Many people still bear emotional scars from disheartening experiences in their youth, such as growing up with authority figures, even parents, who wounded their self-esteem and body image; or having run-ins with physical education teachers who made them feel ungainly and uncoordinated. If that's your situation, then there's a substantial obstacle in your path. Likewise if you're still suffering from a physical or psychological trauma that happened long ago but that you've never adequately addressed. Divorces, family fights, loneliness, grief, a sense of purposelessness—these are all things that can be significant barriers to successful weight loss. When someone is inactive and overeats, it frequently gets chalked up to laziness and lack of willpower, but more often than not, the real reasons that someone can't muster up the motivation are far more complex.

While I love the work I do, one thing I don't like about the diet-and-fitness industry in general is that the psychological side of weight loss—and its importance—is rarely fully acknowledged. Instead, much of the industry seems to thrive on hooking people on the diet and exercise plans du jour, each one hawked as a breakthrough. My problem with these plans is that they lead people to believe (or they even say outright) that if you *just* eat some magic combination of food or work out in some special way, you will lose weight and keep it off forever. In fact, we now have pretty good data showing that one program doesn't work all that much better than the next as long as calories are cut and activity is boosted; what matters most is how motivated someone is to stay on a program of reduced calories and increased exercise.

I've always resisted giving the impression that there's any magic to weight loss, or that it's easy. That's another flaw I see in the diet and fitness industry. Weight loss is often presented as something that anyone can do, and with minimal effort. If that were true, there wouldn't be, by some estimates, less than a 20 percent success rate. As they say, the numbers don't lie. That isn't to say that you can't be a part of that successful 20 percent. I want you to be, I encourage you to be, and I know that if you're committed, you will be. But I also know that it requires taking a good, hard look at yourself and your motivations, your triggers, your fears, and your self-talk. You've got to explore and acknowledge your thoughts and feelings, including those that you may have been disregarding for quite a while. Your goal should be to change what's going on inside you. When that happens, changing your eating and exercise habits—and attaining a healthy body weight—will naturally follow.

The emotional and psychological side of weight loss has always been important to me. In previous books of mine, I've even given readers "assignments" to help them get to know their state of mind better. Now I want to take it to a deeper level, and for that I've turned to Ann Kearney-Cooke, PhD, for her expertise. Ann is a psychologist and leading expert in the area of body image and weight control. As director of the Cincinnati Psychotherapy Institute and a distinguished scholar for the Partnership for Women's Health at Columbia University, Ann brings a wealth of both scientific knowledge and hands-on experience to the table. Not only is she familiar with the research in this area, she has spent years working with patients who seek solace and stress relief in food and whose efforts to make healthy changes have been hobbled by low self-esteem or a distorted body image. Talking to people struggling with their weight every day has given Ann considerable insight into the mental and emotional roadblocks standing in the way of success, and has helped her develop effective tools for knocking down those obstacles. Now, in this book, she's going to share them with you.

I have also asked Janis Jibrin, MS, RD, to weigh in on the psychological, physiological, and practical issues that surround overeating and poor food choices. Janis is a Washington, DC–based dietitian who, in her private practice, specializes in weight loss and eating disorders. She is not only well acquainted with the triggers of emotional eating, she is well armed with sensible advice on how to eat more healthfully without completely denying yourself the pleasurable aspects of food. Janis is one of the best dietitians I've ever worked with. She really knows the research, and she has a knack for translating it into workable solutions for people who've tried more than a few times yet failed to lose weight.

Together Ann, Janis, and I are going to give you the tools you need to begin the hard work of change. What we're presenting is an integrated approach to achieving the most fulfilling life possible. Too often people focus on only one aspect of weight loss, be it diet, or exercise, or the psychological aspects of overeating. But that's like fixing only one leg of a table when all of them are wobbly; eventually the other legs are going to give out, and the table is going to collapse even if the strong leg holds steady. Being overweight tends to be a multifaceted problem. We're going to help you tackle it from every angle, and that includes strengthening your emotional foundation as well as dealing with the physiological hardwiring we all have that further complicates our efforts to change. Many people who don't triumph at weight loss beat themselves up without taking into consideration that humans are predisposed to eat as much fat and sugar as possible to conserve our energy and to avoid discomfort—all of which contribute to the difficulty of changing eating and exercise habits. The truth is, there are some things about your physiology that you can't change, and a natural propensity to seek pleasure is one of them.

What you can change, however, is what gives you pleasure as well as your tolerance for discomfort.

The majority of people who succeed at weight loss have the same built-in inclinations and susceptibilities as you; they've simply been able to overcome them or at least manage them. And not because they're superhuman. Most of them have successfully changed what gives them pleasure and increased their tolerance for discomfort because they've changed the most important thing of all: *their minds.* They think differently now about what it takes to reach weight loss goals. If they once may have believed that success was all about transforming their bodies with diet and physical activity, they know now that it's really much more about transforming their lives. To obtain a healthier weight, you must, of course, change your eating and exercise habits—that's a given. But the newer and more effective approach to obtaining a healthier weight entails changing your attitudes *and* the way you live.

Earlier I mentioned several of the things that can stand in the way of weight loss, such as unfulfilling jobs, family dramas, and emotional scars, to name just a few. These are issues far more serious than a weakness for desserts, so you can see that clearing the hurdles they present may take some major life renovations. Your relationship with your significant other, your work, financial issues, friendships, priorities—and especially the way you view and treat yourself—may have to change or at least be examined. It's no exaggeration to say that successful losers undergo a true transformation, one that ranks up there with other biggies, such as the transition from childhood to adulthood, from single person to spouse, from dependent student to independent breadwinner.

Ann, Janis, and I have all observed this phenomenon time and time again, and we're not alone. It's also one of the findings of a landmark study called the National Weight Control Registry (NWCR). Some of the most interesting and valuable knowledge those of us in the health field have gained about weight loss comes from the NWCR, a project begun back in 1994 by two researchers, one from the University of Colorado and one from Brown University. Since then, those researchers and their colleagues have collected information on more than six thousand people who've met the enrollment criteria: a loss of at least thirty pounds maintained for one or more years. (The average weight loss among the participants is actually sixty-six pounds, maintained for an average of five and a half years; some of them have even kept their weight off for more than sixteen years!)

There are many things that have helped the NWCR participants prevent weight regain. I will fill out the picture for you in a later chapter, but in the meantime, I think it's important to know at the outset of your own journey that transformation played a critical role in their success. "Radical weight loss without a newly defined identity is impossible to maintain, as massive evidence has shown in countless research studies, including the NWCR," says Inga Treitler, PhD, a cultural anthropologist who has spent intense one-on-one time documenting the lives of NWCR participants. "This new identity requires letting go of part of the old life and adopting new habits that fit with the transformed identity."

In my own observations, I've seen that sometimes the transformations are small: the guy who gives up a life in front of the TV to go out and play baseball with his son, the woman who skips enchiladas and margaritas with the gals to work out at the gym, the couple who replace their drinking buddies with walking buddies. And sometimes the transformations are radical. There's the workaholic who switches (and downsizes) careers, the mom who confronts and ultimately spends less time with family members who are sabotaging her efforts to improve her health, and the people who even go so far as to end a relationship in order to better their lives.

Years ago, I met a man at my gym—call him John—who was worried about his wife—let's refer to her as Denise—a woman both overweight and unhappy. I was already overbooked at the time, but this man's genuine concern for his wife made me decide to free up time for an initial consultation with Denise. She ended up becoming a regular client.

Denise slowly started dropping weight, but she still seemed just as unhappy as when we'd started. The more I worked with her, the clearer it became why: Although she cared for John, he was holding her back in many ways, not the least of which was from pursuing her dream of acting. What's more, while John had engaged me to help Denise, the closer she got to her goal weight, the more threatened he became by her newfound confidence and determination. Their marriage obviously wasn't working for many reasons, these being just two of them. I knew that Denise would have to address the problems in her marriage if she ever wanted to reach her goal weight and live a happy life, and eventually she did. Denise and John divorced, and shortly thereafter, she landed the lead in a play—her lifelong dream. Through her work on the stage, she met the man of her dreams, also an actor, whom she later married.

A cautionary tale? Yes and no. I'm not saying that divorce is the answer to all of life's problems. In Denise's case, her strained marriage was preventing her from realizing her dreams and living a happy and fulfilled life. Is something preventing *you* from realizing your dreams and living a happy and fulfilled life? Realizing what changes you need to make and actually acting on them can be hard, even painful. But the results—happiness, joy, confidence, a renewed sense of self, to name just a few—are more than worth it.

HOW THIS BOOK WORKS

While you'll find practical advice about eating and exercise scattered throughout, this book is really about how to improve your psychological and emotional well-being. It's all about exposing the barriers that not only seem to make it logistically impossible to eat well and exercise but also sap your motivation to do either. This is the book that's going to help you get to the bottom of why you keep starting diet and fitness programs enthusiastically only to lose your incentive and stop (and then start and stop all over again). Or, if you've never gotten started in the first place, this is the book that's going to help you understand why. Everything in these pages is designed to help you attend to what's going on inside you (your mind, your way of thinking) so that you can get on with the business of improving what's on your outside (your body weight). So how do you go about that?

First, I believe it's helpful to look at the big picture. There are many, many obstacles that stand in the way of weight loss, and we'll run through them systematically throughout this book. However, there are also a few common and particularly significant barriers that trip people up. Those barriers range from feelings of unworthiness to sexual abuse. One or more—or perhaps none—of them may strike a chord with you, but whichever it is, reading about these obstacles will get the wheels turning in your head and help you to begin thinking about what in your life is holding you back from success.

The chapters that follow get even more specific and cover six separate but inter-related topics: overcoming overeating, becoming a healthy eater, ending exercise aversion, improving your body image, learning how to maintain weight loss, and pursuing happiness. Whether it's Ann, Janis, or me doing the talking, our goal is the same: to help you take a thorough and honest look at your attitude toward each aspect of achieving your best possible life. I find that most people operate on autopilot, rarely taking the time to be introspective about the reasons they do—or don't do—things. Each chapter is designed to slow you down, help you become more self-reflective, and see yourself in a clearer light. Some of that will come from asking yourself questions. We'll ask you to "interview" yourself to assess how motivated you are to change various aspects of your life. Some of it will also come from reading about different scenarios that prevent people from reaching their weight loss goals—scenarios that I think will sound familiar. When you can recognize yourself in a situation and say, "Hey, that's me!" you're moving toward finding the reason(s) that you haven't been able to lose weight or maintain weight loss in the past.

At points we'll ask you to take stock of what you're eating and how much you're moving, even how many hours of sleep you get, by keeping a detailed log. You may have kept food or exercise logs in the past; this time around we'll guide you on how to best use this valuable information to make significant shifts in the way you act and even think. If you're like most people, you probably dread the idea of logging—but I strongly suggest that you try it, at least for a few days or a week. Study after study proves it and I've seen firsthand with my clients: Logging is an important tool in achieving weight loss success.

While recognizing your personal barriers is half the battle, you'll also need to take practical steps to better your psychological and emotional life. If, for instance, you're stressed at work and at home because you have a lack of boundaries—you take on every office responsibility and household task regardless of the fact that you're overwhelmed—how do you go about creating limits and taking the pressure off yourself? Or, if you hate to exercise (and, in my experience, most inactive people put exercise in the same category as dental work), how do you learn to like it, or at least find a way to endure it? We'll be giving you tangible solutions to these and many other dilemmas that stand in the way of weight loss success.

Soul-searching, which this approach to weight loss requires a lot of, is never easy. But it's almost always productive. It's somewhat like looking at a road map: You need to know where you are before you can determine how to get to where you want to go. Moving forward, though, almost always requires making one or more tough decisions. I've never met someone who's lost weight and kept it off long term who didn't make the choice to change something significant (a job, a relationship, a cherished habit) in his or her life.

There are essentially two ways you can look at the difficulties ahead of you. You can feel put upon and sorry for yourself, angry that life isn't fair, or you can see the challenges that lay before you as an opportunity to alter something about yourself or your situation that you don't like. Which attitude do you think is going to help you get and stay motivated? Embracing the challenges, of course! It's what separates people who succeed from people who don't. While the prevailing sentiment "woe is me" drains motivation, looking at the hurdles you face as a chance to take a new direction in life can give you meaning and purpose and be a powerful motivator. In some ways, you might even consider being overweight a blessing, as it is calling attention to something else that needs to be addressed. Anything that gives you the impetus to make profound changes in your life could be considered a good thing.

Naturally, my goal isn't just to get you to make changes; my goal is to get you to make changes that *last*. It's wonderful if you lose weight, but only if you keep it off. In chapter 6, we'll revisit the National Weight Control Registry. How have the participants in the registry managed to keep off the weight they lost? Once you make the transformation I hope this book inspires you to make, how do you keep from edging back to your old self? I think the lessons learned from successful people will provide some insight into both the practical matters of weight maintenance and what you might call matters of enthusiasm.

Over the last decade, the number one question people ask me is, "How do you *stay* motivated?" It would be nice if I had one answer for everyone, but the truth is that the answer is different for each person. Finding what motivates you is a process that starts with identifying what's important in your life, picturing your life as you want it to be, recognizing the barriers that keep you from having that life, then compiling a plan of action to remove the obstacles standing in your way. You need to know what life you want (as well as what life you *don't* want), then you have to muster up the will and the drive to go after it. Make the tough choices, remove those barriers, and you'll be on your way to living—*really* living the life you want.

1

BARRIERS TO WEIGHT LOSS SUCCESS

By Bob Greene

ON SOME DAYS, MOTIVATION comes easily. You just feel tired of your old life and ready to make a new one for yourself. *Bring on the challenge,* you say to yourself, *I'm ready to go.* Then the next day . . . you aren't. That inspired feeling, that drive to do things differently, has slipped through your fingers like grains of sand. Where did it go? Why do you feel a strong incentive to change one day and so unmotivated the next?

We all have barriers that can get in the way of our success. It's part of the human condition, where nothing is simple and everything is interconnected. Messy thoughts and emotions, complex relationships, deeply imprinted habits, disquieting memories, the demands of a very complicated world—these things all conspire to set up roadblocks that make it difficult to achieve our goals. And when one of those goals is to achieve a healthier weight, our human physiological wiring also gets thrown into the mix, adding another obstacle to success. Once you get fired up about something and want to change, it should be easy to sustain that drive and enthusiasm. It *should* be easy, but there are many, many reasons why it's not.

Those reasons—barriers, as I call them—are at the heart of this book. The following chapters are going to discuss them in detail and, most important, give you direction on how to overcome them. First, though, I'd like to talk about eight of those barriers that I think are particularly significant. Professionals who work in the field of weight loss find that these eight barriers are especially prevalent among people who are on the diet and exercise roller coaster. When someone continually goes on and off weight loss programs, always gaining back the weight that was lost, it's almost certain that one or more of these obstacles are standing in his or her way. And not only do these obstacles derail healthy eating and exercise, they also erode motivation. So even if you start out gung ho for change, it's hard to stay motivated when you are constantly hitting the equivalent of a cement wall.

While we'll be dealing with these eight barriers in considerable depth throughout the book, I want to introduce you to them now to get you thinking about what might be the biggest challenges to your own success, and to prepare you to examine yourself on an even deeper level in the chapters to come. You may find that one or more of these eight barriers apply to you, while some of them do not. At the very least, though, reading through them may help you better grasp the concept of why losing weight isn't just a matter of finding the right diet and exercise plan. A lot of people are quick to blame failure on the diets or exercise programs they've tried, believing that if they could only discover an absolutely spectacular plan, their motivation would never flag and they would achieve long-term weight loss. The truth is, that kind of thinking only distracts you from discovering what's *really* preventing you from achieving a healthier weight, and it keeps you from doing the work you need to do to be successful. Taking an honest look at what you want in life and figuring out what you need to do to get there is a much better way to spend your time—and a much greater predictor of success.

Are you aware of any of the barriers that might have prevented you from losing weight in the past? Some people can accurately name the barriers they face; however, many are completely unaware of their existence. Or they're focusing on the wrong ones. This book is all about helping you find the right ones—the barriers that are affecting you personally. Sometimes you just need someone to hold up a mirror so that you can see yourself better, and that's our aim here. Becoming aware of what's standing in your way is the first step toward surmounting those hurdles.

Almost everyone who has achieved something meaningful has overcome some kind of barrier. It's a powerful experience that changes your life in profound ways. One of the critical differences between people who are successful and those who aren't is that successful people view obstacles as a challenge. Think of basketball great Michael Jordan, who, if you can believe it, was actually cut from his high school basketball team. Albert Einstein was harshly criticized when he first presented some of his ideas, and one of America's most beloved poets, Emily Dickinson, published little in her lifetime and was reviewed unfavorably by critics, but she kept writing nonetheless. There are countless examples of people who have not let setbacks stand in their way.

When you take action to improve your situation and overcome whatever is preventing you from losing weight, you won't end up with just a slimmer body. You will end up with a newfound confidence and drive, an ability to take control of your life and make the things that you want in *all* areas of your life happen. Losing weight, while important, is the least of it. Identifying and overcoming your barriers helps you become not just a physically healthier person but also a psychologically and emotionally healthier person. That's when you're going to be living a much richer and more fulfilling life.

EIGHT SIGNIFICANT BARRIERS TO SUCCESS

Barrier 1: An Aversion to Discomfort and Pain

Like all creatures, we are programmed to move toward pleasure and to avoid pain. It's part of our survival instincts. Let's forget the pleasure half of the equation for a moment and talk about pain—or, really, its somewhat lesser cousin, discomfort. The most obvious things that cause discomfort and make it hard for people to change their eating and exercise habits are (1) the anxiety and dissatisfaction they feel when they are denied foods that their bodies crave with every inch of their being, and (2) the unpleasant (and slightly panicky) feeling that arises during exercise when their breathing accelerates and their muscles begin to throb. *I want the instant gratification of my chocolate muffin. My stomach rumbles if I don't have something to eat before bed. I don't want to feel sweaty or my heart beating against my chest.* Anyone who hates deprivation and physical exertion—and a large number of people do—is going to find it hard to stick to a plan that requires coping with both things regularly.

Everybody, though, experiences discomfort differently, and many people have a higher threshold for discomfort than others. That's one thing that may separate those who are eventually able to lose weight and keep it off from those who can't seem to get it right. But success—or failure—as it relates to discomfort is not quite as simple as that. Eating unhealthfully and avoiding physical activity not only lets people evade unpleasant things like chocolate withdrawal and sweaty gym clothes, it allows them to dodge dealing with uncomfortable emotional pain. For those people, especially if they're emotional overeaters, the biggest barrier to weight loss is an aversion to the pain or discomfort of confronting personal issues.

And yet here is an odd little twist to the whole idea of how an aversion to discomfort and pain can get in the way of long-term weight loss. Angela Taylor, LCSW, a licensed psychotherapist in Los Angeles who specializes in eating disorders and weight management, points out that some people also use something they find painful—say, a feeling of self-loathing and embarrassment about being fat—to motivate them to change their eating and exercise habits. That might sound like a good thing, and it *can* be a good way to jump-start a program, but ultimately it may be impossible to stick with a way of life that is solely driven by such negative feelings. "In most things in life, we use pleasure to motivate us," observes Taylor. "We reward kids with gold stars to motivate them, we give ourselves vacations for a job well done. But somehow, when it comes to weight loss, people seem to be more motivated in the beginning by things that trigger their pain center. And it's typically not sustainable. You burn out because the natural inclination is to run away from pain."

One exception to this viewpoint is the fear of becoming ill—or actually becoming ill. For example, suffering a heart attack (or being told by your doctor that you might if you don't lose weight) or learning that you are prediabetic can be powerful motivators. I've seen many people, roused by illness or a fear of illness, suddenly adopt regular healthy behaviors after years of inconsistency. It can be the most influential motivator there is. Yet in cases where these threats don't exist, pleasure is often a stronger motivator for changing habits. "If you can find a way to introduce pleasure into the experience, it shifts your mind-set," says Taylor.

As it is, many people's minds are closed to the idea that they may find some pleasure in changing old habits, and that's often due to the "stories" they tell themselves about healthy eating and exercise: They expect it to be unpleasant, and so it becomes a self-fulfilling prophecy. Say, for instance, that you start a new job, and your coworkers gossip to you about Gary in the mailroom. "Oh, Gary is so awful." "He has a bad temper." "You're going to hate Gary." By the time you do finally meet Gary, you're going to have him pegged because of all the stories you've heard about him. The poor guy isn't going to have a chance with you.

In the same way, people often tell themselves stories about the gym and nutritious meals, dashing any hope that they're going to find something to like about either. "The brain likes to take shortcuts. It analyzes, compares, and makes associations so that it doesn't have to learn something new in every situation," explains Taylor. "So if you associate the gym with pain, pretty soon just pulling into the parking lot or looking at your gym clothes is going to stir up feelings of dread. Your brain skips the middle part, so that pretty soon you only have to look at your gym clothes, and your mind thinks, *Ugh*."

The good thing about the brain, though, is that it's malleable. You can learn new, more pleasant associations, even if you have to consciously think about what those pleasant associations are: "The gym gives me a break from my family." "I feel calmer after I've gone out for a brisk walk." "If I don't eat so much at dinner, my clothes don't feel so uncomfortable." And so on. In subsequent chapters, we'll be dealing a lot with how to zero in on the pleasurable aspects of healthy living. If the barrier that's stopping you is an aversion to discomfort, that's going to help you move closer to success.

Barrier 2: Caught Up in the Business of Life

Our culture dictates that the more we do, the more we will get out of life. In response to this, many people work too much, commit to too many activities—and even overschedule their kids. Yet instead of feeling fulfilled and contented, they end up stressed, exhausted, and *hungry*. Your true hunger for rest, meaning in life, balance, and closeness with others may register as cravings for food and alcohol, and even other things, such as drugs. As the stress of being too busy increases, you can begin to feel out of control.

Being caught up in the business of life can become a huge barrier to success for several reasons. Besides making you hungry in the ways I just mentioned, it gives you the idea that you are too busy to attend to your health. It's your out: "I can't exercise, I can't make healthy meals; my schedule just won't permit it." Yet many busy people do eat right and exercise, and one reason they're able to do it is because they make it a priority. They find balance. But if you're overcommitting in other areas of your life, you're not going to achieve that balance.

People who overbook their lives often have trouble saying no, limiting time with people who stress them out, and letting go of perfectionistic standards for both themselves and others. All these things, too, stand in the way of long-term weight loss success because they make it almost impossible to find the time or an acceptable means of nurturing yourself. But nurturing yourself is not a luxury, it's a necessity. In chapter 4, I'll specifically address the excuse that people often use to avoid exercise: "I don't have time." You'll see that, despite your busy life, you actually can work physical activity and eating nutritiously into your schedule.

LOSING TO GAIN A CAREER DREAM

The signs were all there: the fact that simply turning over in bed made him out of breath, the alarming reflection of his 375-pound body in the mirror, and then his doctor mentioning the words *gastric bypass*. But what finally nudged Shaun Tympanick to do something about his weight was the realization that if he didn't, his career dreams would never come true.

"I'd been a probation officer for years and was sick of it. There were these far more interesting law enforcement jobs I wanted so badly, but at my weight, there was no way I could get through police academy training," explains Shaun, who, like many of the people you'll be reading about throughout this book, is a participant in the National Weight Control Registry. To help him out, his brother bought him a gym membership and they went together. He focused on cardio—the treadmill, bicycle, step machine—and he and his brother became hooked on racquetball.

Meanwhile, he overhauled his diet. "I used to eat out every single night," recalls Shaun. "A lot of it was fast food, which I cut out completely. Somewhere midway through my weight loss, I bit into a chicken nugget and it tasted like bleach. I was relieved; I'd been afraid that even tasting fast food again would make me revert back to my old ways."

Shaun lost 155 pounds in just fourteen months. The first 100 pounds took nine months to lose; five months later, he lost the last 55. For three years, he has been maintaining at 220, which feels just right for his six-foot-three-inch frame. A year later, Shaun entered the police academy. "More than the badge and the gun, I wanted the Physical Training Award. I was the fastest guy there and could outrun anyone on the obstacle course. When the instructor presented me with the award, he couldn't believe that I used to be so completely out of shape."

After graduation, Shaun landed his dream job with the U.S. Department of Homeland Security. "Just because I've met my goals doesn't mean I'm going to slack off," he emphasizes. "I run seven miles straight three or four times a week. Once a year, I guest lecture a high school criminal justice class my brother teaches. I tell the students that you don't just get fit to graduate. God forbid you have to defend yourself on the job— you need to be fit for that." When his coworkers rib him about being a diet and exercise freak, he asks them, "If there's a scuffle or a serious incident, who'd you rather be at your side: the fit guy or the unfit one?"

Barrier 3: Your Pleasure-Seeking Physiological Wiring

Our bodies are incredibly elegant machines. They have wiring, which was laid down about one hundred thousand years ago, that helps us avoid starvation by influencing our food preferences and appetite. That was useful to our cavemen ancestors, but, of course, most of us have little chance of starvation today. In fact, with today's overabundance of food, this hardwiring is more of a liability than an asset.

Everyone's brain is programmed to seek pleasure, a mechanism that encourages us to consume more high-calorie foods. Given the body's drive to store body fat in anticipation of leaner times, every time you munch on a bag of chips or scarf down a doughnut, pathways in your brain trigger the release of neurotransmitters such as endorphins and serotonin, chemical messengers associated with positive emotions. That's why it feels so good. And if you use foods to self-medicate when you feel lonely or sad or stressed, you reinforce the system. The next time you're in the same emotional low, your brain will remember what gave you relief the last time and urge you to eat those chips or doughnuts all over again.

The body's natural propensity for pleasure can be one of the biggest barriers to changing habits. How many times has someone set a piece of cake in front of you and part of your mind tells you "no, no, no" while the other part whispers "yes, yes, yes"? The latter is a tough impulse to fight, especially for some people. Evidence suggests that, while we may all have pleasure-seeking encoding in our brains, overweight people in particular seem to have malfunctions in this system, compelling them to eat more than other people to get the same "buzz" from high-calorie foods.

In chapter 3, Janis is going to sketch out the physiological barriers to weight loss in full, but one thing you should know right off the bat is that the reward centers of the brain—where the pleasure of those high-calorie foods registers—also respond to other substances that bring about pleasure. That's why alcohol, drugs (including the nicotine in cigarettes), and high-calorie food can be equally addicting and why many people begin overeating when they give up those other vices. But those reward centers also respond to other gratifying things, like watching a beautiful sunset or experiencing a loving touch—or the endorphins produced by exercise. So while you may not be able to change the wiring in your brain, you can "feed" those reward centers other pleasures. That's the key to overcoming this hurdle. Biology isn't destiny when you have effective strategies like the ones you'll find throughout this book firmly in place.

Barrier 4: Feelings of Unworthiness

If you ask someone, "Do you feel worthy of having a good life?" that person will almost always answer, "Of course." But is that the truth? Often, when you get down to the specifics of what someone feels he or she deserves in life, the answer is no.

Self-worth is having a sense that it's okay for you to get what you want and to enjoy life. It's also a sense that your opinions, your priorities, and your needs matter as much as the next person's. People who have a sense of unworthiness, on the other hand, may chronically apologize for their actions, find it hard to accept a compliment, let other people take advantage of them, be quick to take the blame for things that aren't even their fault, and sublimate their needs in favor of the needs of others.

Unworthiness interferes with weight loss in a variety of ways. For one thing, adopting healthy habits requires that you put yourself first in many respects. It may mean doing things like choosing to serve lean meats and piles of vegetables instead of the macaroni and cheese that your family prefers; leaving your child with a babysitter or your mom for an hour so that you can go to the gym; or putting the brakes on overtime so that you can get enough sleep even though your coworkers are staying late. People who don't have a healthy self-worth don't take these necessary steps. They are doormats, worried that their actions of self-love (or even just self-preservation) will hurt or inconvenience someone else. They find it all too easy to defer to everyone else, which makes it very hard to concentrate on developing healthier habits for themselves.

Unworthiness can also be an obstacle to living up to your full potential if it involves constantly comparing yourself to others and never coming out ahead. If John always gets out and jogs three more days than you, and your colleague Betsy is so strong willed that she never takes even a single bite of cake at office celebrations, you may constantly feel discouraged by your inability to keep up. Again, that's not exactly a good incentive for someone who wants to make big changes in his or her life.

Our sense of self-worth is generally developed when we are children. As Angela

RAISING SELF-WORTH, LOWERING EMOTIONAL EATING

"When I was growing up, there weren't many overweight kids," recalls Cindy Heiss, PhD, RD, a registered dietitian and professor of nutrition at Metropolitan State College of Denver. "I was a little chubby, and I remember getting teased about it on the school bus at age eleven. That's when I went on my first diet." Going from one popular diet to the next, Cindy's weight yo-yoed throughout high school, college, and grad school. At age twenty-five, she lost over 100 pounds on a liquid diet, only to gain it all back, peaking at 258 pounds by age thirty-nine. "I had a PhD in nutrition; I knew people were baffled and extra judgmental about my weight," she reflects. "I felt tremendous shame, which led to a desperation to lose weight quickly and going on weight loss regimens I knew weren't healthy."

Cindy's turning point came a few years later when she caught one of my appearances on Oprah's show in January 2003. "Years before, I'd read Bob and Oprah's book, *Make the Connection,* and realized I was an emotional eater, but I didn't like myself enough then to do anything about it. It wasn't until I heard Bob talk about it on the show that I really internalized it. It hit me that as an emotional eater, dieting wasn't going to work for me; that I was going to have to change the way I lived my life. I realized that I needed to have enough self-worth to take care of myself and that the weight wasn't the primary issue. So on that day, at 258 pounds, I stopped being the 'fat girl' and starting feeling like an inherently worthy person," she says.

Taylor explains, "Watch a small child and you will hear him repeatedly say, 'Look at me, Mommy!' or 'Watch this, Daddy.' In essence, he is saying, 'Am I okay?' When a child receives the message 'Yes, I think you are great,' they feel validated. When they don't, they often develop the habit of thinking of themselves as 'not okay,' and believing they always must 'do better' in order to be 'okay.' This leads to a chronic feeling of unworthiness."

Other things can also lead to low feelings of self-worth. People who get caught up

Eventually, with the help of a nutrition counselor whom she saw not for the nutrition advice but for the support in giving her permission to make herself a priority, Cindy started changing the way she lived. Her first step, literally, was to do something she loved: walking on the beach. On one of those walks, a young man called out, "Look at the beached whale!" Her response: "Instead of thinking I was a defective person, like I did that day at age eleven on the school bus, my first thought was, *What a jerk.*" She also left her exceedingly stressful professorship at a California university for a saner position at a midwestern school. Better eating habits followed, along with a 115-pound weight loss. Now forty-seven years old, Cindy has maintained her weight at around 145 pounds—a comfortable size 8—for more than five years.

How did she stop using food to cope? "I've had to learn to take better care of myself, which involved learning to say no," she explains. "That was tough. I had to overcome a victim-martyr mentality and realize that I had a choice in how to live my life. Putting myself first was—and still is—hard. I'm a perfectionist who tries too hard to be liked by everyone, which is impossible, and I have to force myself not to work too hard."

Cindy still gets the urge to overeat when she's very stressed, but she reminds herself that "my problems won't be solved by a bowl of ice cream." Instead she now copes by exercising, going to the gym, or taking a walk in the park, and by contacting friends. "My best friend is my sister; we talk at least every other day. I also joined a women's support group in Denver that meets once a week—that helps me develop further insight and provides tremendous support—and I rely on other friends as well," says Cindy. "Before, it was hard for me to ask for help; now it's getting easier."

in the media images surrounding us—the perfect bodies, the airbrushed faces—may feel insignificant by comparison because they can't match those images. (Who can?) People who feel guilty for something, real or imagined, that they did may also feel they don't deserve a better life. Often, children of physical or sexual abuse grow up believing that they did something wrong and therefore brought on the abuse. And the abuse itself reinforces the fact that they're unworthy of love and respect; why else would someone treat them that way? Those feelings of guilt and/or low self-worth can get carried into adulthood, making a person feel undeserving of any of the good things in life.

Unworthiness can be a deeply held belief, and getting past it involves a lot of self-examination. But just identifying the problem can be liberating. Once people with low self-worth begin looking at their *real* value to others, it becomes easier for them to appreciate themselves. "They also see that you don't have to be like the people at the other end of the spectrum—people who value themselves so much that they are selfish and literally railroad others to get what they want—to have a healthy sense of self-worth," says Taylor. "There is a middle ground where you feel as though you are allowed to have what you need and know that you can get it without hurting other people."

Barrier 5: Fear of Success (or Failure)

In some ways, it doesn't seem to make sense: If you want to lose weight, how could you possibly be *afraid* of losing weight? Yet many people *are* afraid of successfully slimming down, even if they don't realize it. Sometimes this fear harks back to barrier 4: feelings of unworthiness. "I call it the Swiss cheese phenomenon," says Ann Kearney-Cooke. "If your core belief is that you are not worthy of success, everything positive that happens to you falls through the holes of the cheese, while everything negative sticks. You get used to the core belief that you shouldn't succeed; it's where you feel safe."

People who are afraid of losing weight may fantasize about changing their bodies, but the reality of that change can be unsettling. Weight loss is a very visible way to take control of your well-being. If you're depressed and get better, very few people are going to notice and comment on your improved health. But, let's face it, friends, family, and even acquaintances love to commend weight loss. Even if their observations are complimentary—"You look fabulous!"—the attention can be embarrassing and make you feel as though your privacy has been invaded.

Some people also fear that weight loss will shake up the status quo in ways they may not be able to handle. If, for instance, you use food to cope, knowing that you can no longer turn to a pint of ice cream after, say, a bad day at work can provoke anxiety about how you're going to deal with stressful or chaotic episodes in your life. Weight loss can change the dynamics of a marriage, too: not only because the other spouse may feel threatened now that his or her partner is more attractive to outsiders but also because it requires a new, healthier way of living that he or she finds unacceptable. Anyone at all apprehensive about upsetting the apple cart in a relationship is a perfect candidate for feeling afraid of change. The fear may be unconscious, yet if it's there, quietly nibbling at your brain, it's going to be a barrier to achieving your goals.

Fear of success is often common in people who have had a history of sexual abuse. For them, the kind of attention I mentioned earlier can be embarrassing and, worse, feel threatening. Ann had a client (see page 61) who had been abused as a child and struggled with her weight as an adult. The woman was eventually able to drop a significant number of pounds, getting down to a size 10. "One day, she went to the mall, and she had a paranoid, uneasy feeling as she was getting out of her car," recalls Ann. "Then a man opened the mall's door for her, and she could feel him noticing her body. It made her feel unsafe." There's no doubt that a bigger body is easier to hide behind, and many people sabotage their own weight loss efforts for that very reason. For them, fear of successful weight loss is really fear of sexual vulnerability. "When my client was little, she wasn't safe," observes Ann, "but as a grown woman, she now had the skills to handle unwanted attention. I had to remind her that she wasn't vulnerable anymore."

The flip side to fear of success is fear of failure. To be honest, there is some logic to this fear. The data indicate that most people do fail at long-term weight loss. And if you're like most people, maybe you've already been through several cycles of success-fully shedding pounds only to regain them all (and sometimes even more). But I think it can also be said that you shouldn't let past failures or the failures of the population at large worry you. For one thing, most people don't keep off the weight the first time; it can take a few rounds before you learn from your mistakes and figure out what will and won't work for you personally. For another thing, this book is going to help you take a holistic approach to weight loss. In the past, you may have addressed weight loss from only one angle—just as many of the people who end up as failure statistics do. As I outlined in the introduction, we're going to help you deal with the emotional-psycho-logical side of weight loss in combination with the practical eating and exercise issues. That kind of integrated approach is going to greatly increase your odds of success.

Barrier 6: A Poor Body Image

Body image is best described as the picture that someone has of his or her body and the thoughts and feelings associated with it. How you feel about your body influences every aspect of your life: your self-esteem, your mood, and, by extension, your overall health. In a way that is similar to feelings of unworthiness, a negative body image can make you feel unworthy of achieving the "good life"—complete with healthy relation-ships, a great job, a loving family, and fun hobbies—and rob you of the motivation to change your lifestyle.

Many factors determine body image. It can have to do with whether you were teased about your body as a child and whether your parents either praised or criticized your shape and weight. It can also be determined by how your parents talked and felt about their own bodies. Traumatic events such as sexual or physical abuse can also influence body image, as can the culture we live in. Living in a culture obsessed with thinness makes it difficult to navigate life as an overweight person and hard to cope with weight-related stigma and discrimination. Many overweight people internalize these prejudices and negative stereotypes, which can further contribute to a negative body image and low self-esteem.

Part of the mission of this book is to help you develop a different type of relationship with your body. It's crucial to not only accept your body but also make taking care of it a priority, no matter what else is happening in your life. "You might worry, 'If I accept my body, then I will become complacent and just gain more weight,'" says Ann. "However, I have found that the opposite is true: Beating yourself up about your appearance and putting yourself down is the *last* thing that motivates healthy lifestyle change." In fact, once you are able to improve your body image, you will choose to actively take care of your body (by, say, increasing your physical activity, and giving up fried foods and overeating at night). What's more, you'll insist that those around you treat your body with respect, removing another barrier to long-term weight loss. It's challenging to lose weight without the understanding and sometimes even the help of family, friends, and coworkers. When you let them know that you are serious about treating your body right, chances are they'll fall in line too.

Check out the body image chapter in this book. It's filled with strategies that'll help you let go of a negative body image and develop a positive, healthy one instead.

Barrier 7: Unsupportive Relationships with Adults When You Were Young

I'm not a psychologist, but sometimes when I'm working with clients, trying to probe a little bit about why sticking to a fitness program has been difficult for them, they talk to me as though I am. And I've been surprised at how many of those clients end up talking to me about their early lives and the expectations placed on them by their mothers or some other authority figure. It's not uncommon for people to still harbor hurt feelings and fears well into adulthood, and for those feelings and fears to have a profound impact on their motivation to exercise and ability to control their eating.

It's a topic of fascination to me, and I asked Angela Taylor about it. She, too, has many clients who eventually bring the conversation around to Mom or Dad, an older sibling, or a teacher when trying to understand their reasons for not being able to lose weight. As Taylor explains it, a lot of that has to do with how our brains form connections when we're young.

"When we're kids, every experience creates neuroconnections—sort of like grooves—in our brains and impacts the level of safety we feel, if our needs are being met, if we're stimulated. At the same time, thoughts, emotions, and beliefs are getting tied into these neuroconnections. Now fast-forward to when we're adults, and if anything happens to us that is related to our experience as a child, it fires up the old neural pathways as though we were that age all over again."

Say, for instance, that your mother told you to stop eating so much or you would get fat. Or your older sister once said you were fat and nobody was going to like you. Or you loved dance and thought you were beautiful until your dance teacher poked your belly and said you were never going to make it in dance. With your adult brain, you could probably handle these discouraging but not necessarily devastating verbal jabs. "But to your eight-year-old brain, they're traumatizing," says Taylor, "and when something brings you back to those experiences, you operate with your eight-year-old brain, not your adult brain."

In theory, we should have all separated from these early experiences, but as Taylor points out, our brains have long memories. Many adults are still rebelling against the parent, sibling, or teacher who was unsupportive, or have feelings of anger or fear that get triggered every time they try to change their eating and exercise habits. Yet these same people often aren't aware that their current struggles are related to psychological injuries they received in their youth.

Recognizing that you may be acting with your eight-year-old brain can help you make sense of behavior that your logical adult brain has never quite been able to comprehend. "Many people don't understand why they feel so out of control with food; they say, 'It doesn't make sense,'" says Taylor. "But when they realize that it's rooted in early experiences with caregivers, it starts to become clearer."

Barrier 8: Abuse

According to the U.S. Department of Health and Human Services, over 770,000 confirmed cases of child abuse and neglect occur each year. That's an astounding number. Abuse permeates our society, occurring in millions of homes across the country, regardless of class, race, socioeconomic status, religion, or profession. The effects of abuse may not be immediately visible, but they can affect a person for the rest of his or her life. The magnitude of this effect depends on the nature and circumstances of the abuse, the personal temperament of the child, the child's home environment, and the support received after the abuse has taken place.

When an adult—whether it be a parent, caretaker, teacher, relative, or religious figure—who is supposed to love and protect children instead betrays and uses them, their young victims may ask themselves, "What's wrong with me that they did this?" or "How can I ever trust anyone if those closest to me took advantage of me?" Abuse typically can cause self-esteem to plummet and feelings of shame and fear to take root.

In one long-term study, researchers found that, by age twenty-one, as many as 80 percent of young adults who had been abused met the diagnostic criteria for at least one psychiatric disorder, such as depression, anxiety, or suicidal behavior.

I've already mentioned a few times how abuse is linked to some of the barriers to weight loss (for example, feelings of unworthiness and fear of success), but there are also other ways that abuse can present an obstacle to attaining a healthier body and body image. In Ann's work, she has observed a link between childhood abuse and eating disorders. "About one-third of the patients I treat for eating disorders have a history of sexual abuse," she says. "Victims of abuse often feel as though they can't control their bodies and lives. This may lead to lifelong attempts to regain control of their bodies by controlling their weight—either through restriction, obsessive monitoring, and various weight loss strategies or through overeating and chronic obesity. Victims may engage in extreme dieting, starving, bingeing and purging, crash dieting, and detoxes in an attempt to get rid of fat."

But severe restriction never works for long, and many people with abuse in their past end up bingeing: eating large amounts of food, sometimes to the point that they are physically in pain, perpetuating the cycle. They often end up losing and regaining hundreds of pounds during their lifetimes, unable to ease the discomfort of feeling out of control.

Some victims of abuse cope in other ways; they may be more comfortable carrying extra weight as a means to keep others at a distance. They learned that people are toxic, dangerous, and could take advantage of them at any time. As a result, they layer themselves in extra weight, which mimics a space suit or coat of armor around the body, signaling others to stay away. Although they feel unattractive and often wish they could

SHEDDING THE WEIGHT TO COME OUT OF HIDING

At age thirty-two, Mary Jo Schneider carried 300 pounds on her five-foot-four frame. She'd been gaining weight since age nineteen, when, pregnant and alone, she fended off an attempted rape. "I think I was subconsciously using the fat as padding to protect myself and feel safe after that incident," says Mary Jo, now an adult education teacher living in California, and a member of the NWCR. "Plus, I used food to cope with the trauma and with the stress of being a single mother. Food was so soothing."

Mary Jo's scale went up and down for nearly two decades; she hit her lowest weight, 130 pounds, at thirty-five, then packed on 125 pounds by age forty-four. Now sixty years old, she has maintained her weight at 155 pounds for eight years. "There are still days when I use food to cope with emotions," she reflects. "However, now I recognize this as a barometer that something's up that needs my attention, and I address it right away." Her biggest source of support: Overeaters Anonymous peer support groups. "I love OA because it's a spiritual program; it's the root of joy and peace in my life."

lose weight, they are frequently unaware of the strong connection between their past childhood trauma and their current destructive behavior patterns.

The body is where child abuse often occurs, whether the violence is sexual or physical. Sometimes, though, child abuse can also be emotional—for instance, being chronically yelled at by an alcoholic parent or forced to live a life of severe deprivation out of sheer cruelty. "Either way," says Ann, "children who live through abuse have their souls injured, violated, and compromised."

Ann will talk more about the link between abuse and overeating in chapter 2, but if what you've read so far resonates with you, even if it happened years and years ago, it's important to know that this might not be something you can or should handle alone. Because the problem is so widespread, there are therapists all over the country who are well trained to handle the ramifications of abuse. Your number one priority shouldn't be your weight; it should be to deal with any issues that linger from any mistreatment you've suffered, whether it happened when you were a child or as an adult. Once you do that, a healthy weight will likely follow.

2

OVERCOMING EMOTIONAL EATING

By Ann Kearney-Cooke

IT HAS BEEN MONTHS since your divorce. After a quiet weekend, you find yourself at the cupboard mindlessly noshing on chips. You aren't really hungry, but you feel empty and lonely. As you fill up on the chips, you're probably not even aware that you're actually trying to fill an emotional void in your life.

Or it's nine o'clock in the evening, and you've been running around all day hoping to get an impossible number of tasks done. You turn on your favorite television show and begin to eat the pizza just delivered to your apartment, even though you finished dinner only about an hour ago. In your life, as in your meals, you've put "too much on your plate" or "bitten off more than you can chew."

Or perhaps you've just hung up the phone after another particularly stressful fight with your mother or spouse—over your relationship, your job, money, or some other hot-button issue. Instead of reflecting on the argument and digging into your feelings, you grab a spoon and dig into a carton of ice cream. You stuff down your emotions as you stuff yourself.

Maybe you can identify with one of the scenarios above, or perhaps your experiences are slightly different. The list of reasons why we misuse food is endless, and what triggers overeating can vary greatly from person to person. In this chapter, I'll be talking specifically about overeating as a result of emotions. It's important to note that overeating and emotional eating are closely linked, but they're not exclusively related. Emotional eating (any eating that we do to relieve or soothe emotions, such as boredom, anger, or loneliness) often leads to overeating (eating more food than your body needs), but it's possible to eat for emotional reasons without overdoing it. For instance, you may feel stressed and reach for a candy bar or a piece of cake and then feel better; so while you did react to the emotion by eating, you didn't really overeat. Likewise, you can overeat for reasons other than emotions. Our physiological wiring, our environment (things like lighting, music, and even who we're dining with), and even the portion of a particular food doled out on the plate can all lead us to overeat.

The simple fact is that we're all vulnerable to overeating for emotional reasons. Using food as a reward, distraction, comforter, friend, mood booster—basically, any reason other than to satisfy true physical hunger—is something we all learn to do at an early age, and over the years, it becomes ingrained in us. Truthfully, it doesn't really matter how long you've been dealing with emotional eating. Whether you've been battling it since childhood (these are often the toughest cases, but still treatable), or it stems from an adolescent trauma, or it's a more recent problem (you got married or had children and picked up the habit as a coping mechanism for some of life's new stresses), rest assured that you *can* change your behavior. You have the ability to stop misusing food—and this book is going to help you tap into that power.

Successfully switching over to healthy coping mechanisms won't be easy, but it is doable. A key to this process is understanding that if you're an emotional eater, your relationship to food mirrors your relationship to people, including yourself. For instance, in the first example with the chips on the previous page, your heart's hunger for companionship manifests as your stomach's hunger for food. In the second case, the parallel takes on a different form. Not setting limits with others or setting excessive expectations for yourself translates into not respecting the boundaries of your physical fullness. Basically, if you can't say no to people, you can't say no to food, regardless of whether you're actually hungry or not. And if you deny your own needs in order to keep others happy or avoid conflict, as illustrated by the third example, you are apt to compensate by overeating. In order to develop a healthy relationship with food, you have to change not only the way you deal with your emotions but also the way you relate to *others*.

If you're feeling guilty, embarrassed, or ashamed about your emotional eating habit and how it has affected your life, you shouldn't. Most Americans struggle with some form of this problem: Three-quarters of American women ages twenty-five to forty-five report disordered eating (emotional eating is considered disordered eating) and body image dissatisfaction; and 10 percent meet the criteria for clinical eating disorders, according to researchers from the University of North Carolina at Chapel Hill. (Disordered eating is a subclinical eating disorder; people with disordered eating display some irregular eating behaviors but do not suffer the full range of psychological traits usually associated with a full-blown clinical eating disorder.) These stats may provide you with some degree of relief; it can be a comfort to know that many people are dealing with some of the same issues as you are. But don't let this information make you complacent—you'll never be able to get your weight in check and live a healthy and fulfilled life until you can break the spell that food has over you.

To do that, you'll have to embark on a life-changing journey. This might sound intimidating, but don't be overwhelmed; you'll find lots of great advice and techniques in this chapter and throughout the book. Plus, you have the power to make these important changes. Before we begin, let's take a closer look at what emotional eating is and how it develops. Understanding these factors can help you tease out your specific issue(s) and work toward resolving it.

EMOTIONAL EATING: USING FOOD TO COPE

For emotional eaters, food can become a quick fix that distracts attention from deeper issues that are festering inside. Unresolved problems at work, in your marriage, and with other family members or friends can trigger emotional eating. Financial stress, depression (see page 54 for more on depression), boredom, loneliness, body dissatisfaction, fear—these can all lead to emotional eating as well. When you eat for emotional reasons, food becomes your multipurpose elixir, filling you up when and where others have let you down, or making you feel calm and safe. Emotional eating might take the form of a bag of chips from the office vending machine or a few extra cookies after dinner. It could be a full-scale binge (see "The Breakdown of a Binge" on page 71). Or it might be somewhere in between.

You might think that you overeat because you lack willpower, but that's usually not the case. Many outside factors set us up to overeat for emotional reasons, or, at the very least, they feed the problem. Take, for example, our culture. Forget about the fact that there's a fast-food restaurant on practically every corner. Sure, that's an issue, but it's not only that food—particularly fast, cheap, and unhealthy food—is abundant, it's also that time is scarce and effective coping skills are in short supply. We're all stretched to the limit. Perhaps we're caring for our children, who are overscheduled themselves, between all their after-school sports, clubs, playdates, study groups, and more. Maybe we're looking after aging parents. We're responsible for our significant others and our homes. To make matters worse, many of us are working more hours than ever before, leaving us even less time to fit in all of these responsibilities, let alone any extra time to work on fulfilling ourselves. Think about it: When was the last time you sat down to a quiet, leisurely home-cooked dinner with your family? More often than not, we eat in shifts: Your children might eat dinner right before their basketball or soccer game, you may pick up something on the way home for yourself, and your spouse might grab some leftovers once he or she gets home from work.

Family dinner isn't the only victim of our frazzled and fast-paced culture. We're becoming more and more disconnected from one another in general: family, friends, even our neighbors. Not too long ago, our neighbors were almost like an extension of our family. We all knew one another well, looked out for one another, socialized with one another. Now we're lucky if we know our neighbors' names.

But a shortage of time is only partly to blame for this distancing from friends and family. There are other issues at work, too, such as technologies like cell phones and computers. These are supposed to make staying in touch with loved ones easier and more convenient, but they can actually make us more disconnected. Texting and emailing lack the personal, intimate quality of a get-together or even a phone call. So while emailing a photo of your kids to the grandparents who live across the country is good, it's not a replacement for an embrace. It falls way short of the real thing—a face-to-face physical encounter—because in the end, it's just a photo. This distance and disconnection from others can leave us feeling lonely, and many of us turn to food for comfort.

Not to mention, eating is fast, easy, and acceptable—and, temporarily, it works. It makes us feel better and fills us up. Food can provide a much-needed break at the end of a busy day. It may become your only "secure" source of pleasure. Food can even offer a way to deal with positive emotions and situations: Maybe you reward yourself with food for an accomplishment, or it serves as a form of entertainment. You may be conditioned to associate food with happy times and celebrations, occasions where food is served and everyone is having a good time. This is a common occurrence at holidays, but it can unwittingly become a habit. When any of this happens, a critical shift has occurred: Food is not simply food anymore. It's your constant companion. It's both predictable and safe; you know for certain that the sweetness or saltiness of each bite will hit your tongue and the sensation of comfort will envelop you. David Thompson,* a thirty-five-year-old single carpenter who struggles with emotional eating, says, "After a tough day when I am frustrated, food is the only thing I look forward to. I eat a large meal, watch my favorite TV shows, and then I start to feel relaxed and sleepy."

Food helps boost your mood and relieve anxiety because it temporarily changes the chemical balance in the body. You may choose to fill up on food loaded with

---

*Names of all Ann Kearney-Cooke's patients in this chapter and in chapters 5 and 7 have been changed to protect their privacy.

sugar, in particular, because eating carbohydrate-heavy foods boosts levels of sero-tonin, a brain chemical that regulates mood. Some foods increase levels of another brain chemical, endorphins, which in turn creates a sense of contentment and emo-tional balance.

Unfortunately, these good feelings don't last. Every emotional eater knows the dark side of using food to cope; there's weight gain, shame, and increasing feelings of hopelessness and failure. The first step toward breaking this cycle is to identify your triggers. You might already have an idea of what yours are, or you might need a little help figuring it out—the Lifestyle Log (appendix 1) is a good place to start. Reviewing some of the more common barriers to overcoming emotional eating (starting on page 48) and using some of the exercises in this chapter can also help clue you in.

If you've kept a log in the past and it has been helpful, then you know why it's so important to record. If you're thinking "been there, done that, and it didn't help," I'm urging you to try it again. This time, try not to think of it as a chore or as a reminder of your failures ("I'm so weak for scarfing down those chips"). Instead, use it as an op-portunity to get to know yourself better and to view your behaviors with interest and compassion ("Wow, I must have been really nervous to have devoured that bag of chips without thinking"). In this chapter and in the upcoming ones, we'll help you use the information in your log to free yourself from being ruled by food or from an exercise aversion or other issues standing in your way.

You'll also work on coming up with one or several reasons why giving up emotional eating is important to you. This is critical: You need to believe that overcoming your emotional eating is crucial to your health and well-being. Then you'll check in with yourself to see how ready you are to make important changes to conquer the problem. Finally, we'll start to work on developing strategies that will help you better manage your specific triggers and encourage you to make the switch to healthy ways of coping that don't involve food.

Your first step: Take a look at what you have to gain from changing your behaviors, using the "Why List" on the following page.

FIND YOUR MOTIVATION

You'll be using the following exercises to tap into your intrinsic motivation. Your first task is to review the Why List, which will provide you with one or more motivating reasons to conquer your emotional eating.

THE WHY LIST: TWELVE REASONS TO STOP USING FOOD TO COPE WITH EMOTIONS (PICK AT LEAST ONE)

The brain rewiring involved in tackling emotional eating is hard work, but when you have a deep belief that it's the right thing to do, the going is easier, because motivation hinges on a sincere belief that you'll *benefit* from changing your behaviors and that you're *capable* of making the changes. Just because your doctor, your spouse, your sister, or this book *tells you* to quit using food to cope, it doesn't necessarily mean that *you* truly believe you need to or should. You have to find compelling reasons that resonate *for you.* Check out our reasons in the list below; some might click for you. If we've missed any that are meaningful to you, write them down in the blank spaces at the end of the list. When you feel your motivation start to dip, these are the reasons you'll go back to time and again to regain your resolve:

1. You'll be at a healthier body weight.

2. You'll have a better lab report. Binge foods are notoriously high in sugar and fat; when you put a lid on them, you'll most likely lower your LDL (low-density lipoprotein), or "bad" cholesterol; triglycerides, a heart-harming blood fat; blood pressure; and blood sugar.

3. You'll stop feeling guilty about food.

4. You'll feel better about your body and weight.

5. You'll have more energy.

6. You'll save money.

7. You'll be a good role model for your children, your spouse, your friends, your coworkers, or someone else.

8. You'll feel more in control over your life.

9. You'll feel a sense of accomplishment.

10. You'll respect yourself and take your needs seriously.

11. You'll be able to really enjoy food as food.

12. You'll not only develop more effective ways of coping with feelings, stress, and relationships, you'll have a better understanding of them as well.

Add your own reasons here:

13. _____

14. _____

15. _____

ASSESS YOUR READINESS FOR (AND RESISTANCE TO) CHANGE

You want to put an end to emotional eating, but how ready are you to change? That's what the following questions, referred to by psychologists as the motivational interview, will assess. This self-evaluation serves a dual purpose: In addition to showing you how prepared you are to change, it also presents a picture of how your life might improve as you stop using food to cope. The motivational interview has become an important tool for psychologists helping clients make difficult changes, such as ending alcohol or drug abuse, or losing weight.

Our twist on this tool is that you're acting as both therapist and client. You'll question yourself without being judgmental and answer honestly. As therapist, feel free to ask yourself follow-up questions, especially when you sense resistance to change. For instance, in question 3, if you answer "not at all important," you could follow up with "And why is that?" That's a great way to unearth a barrier that you can start working on. As client, keep an open mind and be willing to change it. For instance, you might have always told yourself, "I freak out when there are no cookies in the house." But answering question 8 with an open mind, you might say, "Well, maybe I could try one night without cookies, or put the cookies in the trunk of my car so they're harder to get."

Write down your answers to the following questions in a notebook or journal. Every so often, go back to the answers to see if you've made progress and to draw inspiration.

ARE YOU MOTIVATED? GAUGE HOW MUCH

1. How is my current weight affecting my life right now?

2. How is my emotional eating affecting my life right now?

3. On a scale of 0 to 10 (with 0 being not at all important and 10 being critically important), how important is it for me to overcome my emotional eating?

4. What kinds of things have I done in the past to break the habit?

5. Which of these strategies worked and which didn't? Why?

6. Some people say that they're divided: They want to stop emotional eating, but part of them doesn't really want to change. Is this at all true for me?

7. On a scale of 0 to 10 (with 0 being not ready at all and 10 being very ready), how ready am I to work on my emotional eating?

8. What could I start doing today or tomorrow to overcome emotional eating (for instance, identify overeating triggers or try healthier coping mechanisms)?

9. What was my life like before I engaged in emotional eating?

10. How much does it worry me that I might return to old patterns of emotional eating once I change them?

11. What makes me feel like I can sustain my progress?

12. What are my hopes for the future if I am able to end emotional eating and/or lose some weight?

13. How would my life be different if I stopped using food to cope and/or lost weight and adopted a healthier lifestyle?

INTERPRETING YOUR ANSWERS

Questions 1 and 2: How is my current weight affecting my life right now? How is my emotional eating affecting my life right now?

Sometimes it takes getting really fed up with feeling paralyzed by your body or your relationship with food to take action and change your situation. Motivation comes from many sources: some positive ("I love going out with friends; it's more enjoyable than sitting at home alone with a big bag of chips") and some negative ("Being overweight and out of shape is causing me more pain than quitting my nighttime eating"). While answering these questions, make a list of the negative consequences of emotional eating; you can return to this list when you need a reminder.

Question 3: *On a scale of 0 to 10 (with 0 being not at all important and 10 being critically important), how important is it for me to overcome my emotional eating?*

If you're an emotional eater, the more importance you place on ending the problem, the more motivated you'll be to do so. So a higher number bodes better for your progress. However, if, even after going through the Why List, you answered this question with a 5 or less, then revisit it after you finish this chapter. And then go back to the question again after you start making some changes. You might find that it takes on more importance with time.

Questions 4, 5, 10, and 11: *What kinds of things have I done in the past to break the habit? Which of these strategies worked and which didn't? Why? How much does it worry me that I might return to old patterns of emotional eating once I change them? What makes me feel like I can sustain my progress?*

In order to stay motivated, you must believe that you have the skills and ability to change your behavior. Psychologists call this "self-efficacy." For instance, most nuclear physicists wouldn't have a clue how to cut and style hair, while most stylists wouldn't have the foggiest idea how to smash an atom. Neither would have a sense of self-efficacy if asked to do the other's job. Fortunately, *everyone* can manage the steps necessary to overcome emotional eating. You will need to set your own pace, and the progress may not happen all at once, but all the abilities required to overcome emotional eating are already inside of you! We're here to give you the tools to tap into them.

Questions 4 and 5 will help you recall what did and didn't work in the past, and questions 10 and 11 will help you ascertain your confidence about moving forward. Even if you stopped emotional eating for only one day, how did you do it? If you've never tried to stop, then think of some other accomplishment—passing a test, teaching your child something, designing your kitchen, completing a project at work, and so on. You used skills such as organization, patience, and perseverance. You might have left your comfort zone and learned new skills. Could you apply those to overcoming emotional eating?

It's natural to worry that you might slip back into old patterns, but put your energy into answering question 11: What makes you think you *can* overcome this problem?

Questions 6, 7, and 8: *Some people say that they're divided: They want to stop emotional eating, but part of them doesn't really want to change. Is this at all true for me? On a scale of 0 to 10 (with 0 being not ready at all and 10 being very ready), how ready am I to work on my emotional eating? What could I start doing today or tomorrow to overcome emotional eating (for instance, identify overeating triggers or try healthier coping mechanisms)?*

Questions 6 and 7 are about readiness to change. *It's okay if you're not gung ho or don't feel up to quitting emotional eating right away.* As long as you acknowledge that it's a serious concern and that you want to take steps toward resolving it, you're on the right track. Question 8 gives you an opportunity to come up with a specific plan. For instance, you could look at your calendar this week and cross out the least important items so that you don't feel so overscheduled and stressed. (Stress is a major trigger of emotional eating; more on this on page 65.) Later in this chapter, we'll give you lots of strategy options; you'll find something you can start doing right away.

Questions 9, 12, and 13: *What was my life like before I engaged in emotional eating? What are my hopes for the future if I am able to end emotional eating and/or lose some weight? How would my life be different if I stopped using food to cope and/or lost weight and adopted a healthier lifestyle?*

Here's where you get to think about all the good things that will come out of changing your behavior. Most people can remember what a normal relationship with food felt like. For some of you, that might have been way back in childhood. Maybe you were at a healthier weight, had more energy, and weren't distressed about emotional eating. Now think of how good you're going to feel when emotional eating no longer has a grip on you. See yourself in your mind's eye and get specific. For instance, if most of your emotional eating happens at night, how will your evenings be different? Think about how nice it's going to feel to not be bloated and overly full, to no longer have to hide your secret habit from your friends or your spouse, to feel more fully in control of your life. Take the time to imagine yourself in this new place in life and savor the great feeling!

KEEPING TABS ON YOUR FOOD INTAKE

Yes, we're going to recommend that you keep a food log as part of your Lifestyle Log (page 229), and before you roll your eyes or turn the page, let me tell you why it's so important. Numerous studies show that keeping a food log—this one simple act alone— helps people to lose weight and to get back on track if their weight starts increasing. Why? For one, you tend to eat less when you know you have to write it down! Also, it's hard to be in denial of your eating behavior when "3 scoops of ice cream" is sitting there in black and white in your log. Another way the log helps you eat better is by showing what you're missing. For instance, if you see that you're falling short on vegetables, you're more apt to start adding them to your diet.

It's also an incredibly useful tool for overcoming emotional eating because it helps you link emotions to eating episodes. That's why the Lifestyle Log has a "Situation/ Emotions" column: You can jot down what you're feeling or what was happening before and after you ate. By writing down your meals and snacks and the circumstances surrounding them, you'll get invaluable information on your particular triggers. Your log will help answer "How much am I eating? What time of day, in what place, and what emotional state am I in when I reach for the chips and candy? What are my emotional eating triggers?" You may discover that it's after a draining conference call with a client that you step out for a Frappuccino and an oversized muffin. Or that at the tail end of a day packed with work and family duties, you take out the cookies. Or you might simply overeat whenever you're alone or feeling lonely.

The day-to-day triggers uncovered by your log, combined with insights into the root issues you'll get from the rest of this chapter, should make it very clear why you're eating for emotional reasons. This knowledge alone will make it easier to extract yourself from the hold of emotional eating.

Before using the log, please read the instructions on pages 229–230. There you'll learn how to fill out the Hunger Scale, a tool used to determine your hunger and fullness levels. In addition, you'll learn why certain factors are included in the log and how many days you should record. Be sure to write down what you eat *immediately* after eating; people tend to underreport their food consumption by up to 40 percent if they wait to log their intake. You have a better chance of accuracy if you log right away.

After completing the log, here's what to look for:

- Eating when you're not hungry. As explained on page 231, a 5 or higher on the Hunger Scale means that you're not physically hungry. According to your log, how many meals or snacks did you begin when you were at a 5 to 10?

- What was going on when you ate without being physically hungry? Here's where you start connecting the dots linking emotions, situations, and eating. For each meal or snack eaten at a 5 or above, look over at the "Situation/ Emotions" column. Where were you? Were you alone? What were you feeling? What happened earlier that day? Was it frustrating, too fast paced, demanding, or even too exciting?

- Hours of sleep. There's a "Sleep" column in the log because lack of sleep can trigger weight gain and is tied to an increased risk for type 2 diabetes (the most prevalent type, which typically appears in adulthood and is often caused by being overweight). Adequate sleep is necessary for the proper balance of the hormones that affect appetite and fat storage, not to mention the fact that being tired may worsen depression or other mood disorders and sap your motivation. When this happens, you take the familiar path of least resistance: using food to cope.

TACKLING YOUR ISSUES

At this point, you may already have an idea as to why you turn to food to handle your emotions. Likewise, you may be aware of some of the obstacles standing in the way of changing your behavior, and to what degree you're ready and willing to change. Here's where we step in: We're going to offer insight into the common barriers to overcoming emotional eating (you may recognize some of these from chapter 1, where we provided an overview of some of the most significant barriers; we'll expand on these and also take a look at a few other barriers below). Even if you think one of the issues doesn't pertain to you, read through it anyway. You might be surprised to see a little of yourself there.

BARRIER: A FEELING OF UNWORTHINESS

Feeling unworthy is one of the deepest and most pervasive forms of suffering in our culture, especially for women. Whether you feel inadequate, unlovable, flawed, or broken, it can be extremely tough to change your life because, in your mind, there's no reason to—you simply don't deserve better. You believe you're not worthy of happiness or joy or love or acceptance. To soothe these feelings, or even to distract your attention from them, you might bury yourself in food. But this only starts a vicious cycle: You feel inadequate, so you eat. Food may help for a short time, but then you feel guilty and flawed, and you berate yourself for being so weak. This only sets you up for another bout of emotional eating.

When it comes to feelings of unworthiness, I typically see two groups of people: those who are more or less aware that this is their issue and those who aren't. For the latter group, it's more of an insidious problem. They may say all the right things—"I deserve to be happy, I want to lose weight, and I'd like to live a healthy life"—but their actions suggest otherwise. For instance, even though you say you'd like to lose weight, do you find that you never have the time to shop for healthy foods or cook nutritious meals because you're too busy driving your children around or taking care of household chores? Do you go on one diet after the next, get close to your goal, and then give up before you can achieve it? Do you consistently find yourself in a relationship that doesn't bring you any joy or satisfaction, yet you never do anything about it? Do you allow yourself to get stuck in jobs that are unfulfilling, even though you say you want to do something meaningful and rewarding with your life? Do your actions fail to reflect someone who genuinely values herself—in short, that you're someone worthy of love, good health and fitness, great relationships, happiness, and a fulfilled life?

These types of behaviors can be a signal that you *do* struggle with feelings of unworthiness. The underlying thought pattern is that you neither expect good things, nor believe that you deserve them. Consequently, you fail to make the time to go to the farmer's market or cook healthful meals. You never try to work on or end an unhealthy relationship. You don't make the effort to update your resume, search for a new job, or even ask yourself what you want to do. You may find excuses—"I'm just too busy" or "Now's not the best time to be looking for a new job"—or perhaps you let other obligations interfere with your goals. Because you don't really believe deep down that you're worthy of happiness and love and good health, you'll never *act* like you're worthy.

In either case, the key to turning things around is to pinpoint the cause of these feelings. Remember, overeating because of emotional reasons is not a character flaw, it's a sign that you're in pain. Figuring out the source of this pain and the resulting feelings of unworthiness is challenging, but it's essential to changing them. Like many emotional problems we experience as adults, this sense of unworthiness probably has roots in your childhood. As children, we were like sponges, adopting many of the beliefs and emotional patterns of our parents, siblings, and friends. We weren't able to think critically or question the core beliefs about ourselves that we internalized through our interactions with those closest to us. So, for example, if your parents were highly critical, set up many unattainable and conflicting expectations, or blamed you for their unhappiness, you may have ended up feeling like something was wrong with you—that you were not good enough, that you were flawed, and therefore unworthy of love and/ or success in life.

Although these core beliefs are often subconscious, they have incredible power over us. They become the filter through which we see, evaluate, and assign meaning to

SELF-WORTH BREEDS SUCCESS

Bill Jenner had lost and regained hundreds of pounds during his fifty years, and he finally came to see me after he'd put back on the fifty pounds he'd lost during the past year. He knew that his problem maintaining was likely a result of his negative feelings about himself. But he needed help changing his core belief that he was unworthy and unlovable.

In therapy, we talked a lot about Bill's childhood. He shared that for as long as he could remember, his parents fought with each other. They never showed affection toward each other or toward Bill and his sister. And he never knew when a fight would break out. They could be enjoying a family dinner, and out of nowhere the shouting and the verbal abuse would begin. His father would accuse his mother of having affairs, and his mother would put his father down for not being more successful and producing the lifestyle he'd promised.

Unfortunately, the anger between Bill's parents would spill onto the kids. They would criticize Bill about his weight, academic problems, and lack of a social life. They often questioned his intelligence and told him that he would never make anything of himself. After years and years of this criticism, he began to internalize these messages, and as a result, Bill was overly critical of and easily disappointed in himself. He had a low tolerance for frustration, gave up easily, and binged on foods—and, later, as an adult, alcohol.

During therapy, Bill came to some important realizations. First, he was able to see that there was nothing inherently wrong with him: All the criticisms he had endured for years really stemmed from his parents' unhappiness in their marriage. He also discovered that the reason he hadn't done well in school was not that he lacked intelligence but that he'd had an undiagnosed case of attention deficit/hyperactivity disorder, or ADHD. And finally, his anxiety and depression were a result of the stress at home, not simply a weakness or character flaw.

all the outside information we receive. They affect the way we think about ourselves, other people, the world, and the future.

How can you tell if you carry these negative core beliefs about yourself? For some people, it will be fairly obvious. Are you quick to criticize yourself or focus on your flaws and failures? What are the words you use when you think of yourself: *Unattractive?*

I encouraged him to challenge the negative thinking that was sabotaging his progress. For example, when he told me that he ran a five-kilometer race before the local Fourth of July parade, I congratulated him. His response: "It wasn't that great. I ran it a minute and a half slower than I usually do."

I told him that I wanted him to follow three steps whenever he found himself speaking or thinking negatively about himself.

Step 1: I wanted him to picture a stop sign and say "Stop!"

Step 2: I wanted him to imagine that someone he loved said that same negative thing about himself or herself. How would he challenge what they'd said? Bill didn't hesitate before answering, "I would tell them it was awesome that they got up on the Fourth of July and ran a 5K."

Step 3: I asked Bill to think of a positive affirming statement that he could say to himself to replace the original negative thought. He responded, "Good for you, Bill! Instead of sleeping in, you got up early and ran the 5K. Your body is getting stronger, and you're looking better every day."

Over the months, Bill practiced challenging his distorted and negative thoughts using this three-step plan, and soon he found it easier to accept the positive things in his life. He allowed himself to get close to his wife and realized his strengths as a manager at work. He developed a healthy sense of entitlement and self-esteem. With weekly psychotherapy, the help of a nutritionist, and daily exercise, Bill was able to lose thirty pounds and keep it off. For the first time in his life, he felt more comfortable in his own skin and worthy of enjoying the good things in life.

Incompetent? Stupid? But for the majority of people who aren't aware, it will take a little more digging. In this case, you may have to pay particular attention to your behaviors in addition to your self-talk. For instance, as I said earlier, you may say, "I'm lovable, I'm worthy," but then you expect—and put up with—people putting you down or feel that everyone's needs should be met before yours. Also think about how you respond when others compliment you or point out your talents and skills. Do you tend to think they feel sorry for you and are just trying to be nice?

If you answered yes to most of these questions, your core belief about yourself is likely that you are inadequate and unworthy of happiness—or that you simply can't achieve it. Fortunately, core beliefs can be changed, although it does take work. To get started, try looking at all the pros and cons of allowing yourself to feel unworthy; doing so can give you the motivation to actually make these changes.

In a journal or notebook, create three columns. Label the left-hand column "Pros," then below it write down how your feelings of unworthiness are *helping* you or others around you. Most likely this will be a very short list, if you can come up with any positives at all. If you *are* able to think of any advantages—maybe your feelings of unworthiness allow you to feel safe and comfortable—jot them down.

Title the middle column "Cons," and make a list of who those feelings are hurting. You could list yourself (again), because being stuck in this place also drains your energy and prevents you from working on your relationships and other problems. Who else? Perhaps your significant other, who may also be feeling mired in an unhappy, unfulfilling relationship; and your children, who are learning from your example.

And in the right-hand column, make a list of the positive changes that will come about from allowing yourself to feel worthy. For starters, you'll be in a better mood and have more energy, which will allow you to address the issues that are preventing you and your significant other from reconnecting. You'll also be a better role model for your children.

Now that you have a good picture of how these feelings of unworthiness may be limiting you and how much better life can be by working to change these feelings, your next step is to start challenging the idea that you don't deserve good things in life. For example, your parents' unhappy marriage had nothing to do with you—rather, it was due to the battle one of your parents had with alcohol and the stress that the condition caused. Or the reason that you didn't get into an Ivy League school and become a doctor wasn't because you were flawed but because your parents' expectations of you never really matched your own dreams or expectations of yourself. You may have preferred to study art or pursue a career in music.

Finally, work on developing an alternative positive belief about yourself. For example, you might say, "I am competent in most areas of my life and am worthy of success and happiness." Then each day, write down evidence supporting your new belief. For example:

"After all the layoffs at my company, I still have a job."

"I signed up with my wife to walk a 5K race in three months."

"My two kids, whom I adore, love me."

"My faith teaches me that the love of God is always with me."

And so on. If you engage in this simple but positive technique each day, you can change the core belief of unworthiness and simultaneously increase your energy and motivation to lose and keep off excess weight.

The exercises in the rest of this chapter can help give you even more insight into your thoughts and beliefs about yourself and empower you to be more supportive and encouraging toward yourself. If you feel you need more guidance or support, I urge you to confide in someone you trust, whether it's a friend, clergy member, or therapist.

BARRIER: EMOTIONAL PAIN

If you're alive, there's no escaping the experience of pain and loss. Some people have more of it, some have less, but emotional discomfort is an inevitable by-product of interacting with the world. You must learn to accept that pain, discomfort, and insecurities are inevitable. During difficult times, say to yourself, "I don't like discomfort, but I can stand it, I can get through it. It won't last forever." Accepting the inevitability of anguish is a critical coping skill. And as contrary as this may seem, you should allow emotional pain and the feelings it triggers to be your teachers. Listen to what they are trying to tell you about your life. You'll probably find that what's been eating at you is the reason you've been eating.

DEALING WITH DEPRESSION

Everyone feels sad once in a while; it's impossible to be happy all the time. We all experience ups and downs, and it's important to accept periods of unhappiness as part of life. But if your low mood lingers day after day, it could signal clinical depression.

Depression is a complicated condition characterized by feelings of sadness, hopelessness, helplessness, stress, lethargy, decreased interest in social activities, and restlessness. It affects twenty million Americans and can occur alongside a variety of medical conditions (such as cardiovascular disease) and psychological disorders (like anxiety disorders), exacerbating these disorders and negatively affecting treatment outcomes. There are varying degrees of the condition, from major depression, the most severe form, to a less debilitating but still serious version called dysthymia. You can also experience depressive symptoms without being diagnosed with clinical depression.

Studies estimate that about 50 percent of Americans with depression don't seek treatment; and of the half that *does* receive treatment, only 21 percent get the *proper* therapies. This a huge problem because untreated depression can affect your relationships, your work, your health, and your weight loss or maintenance efforts. When you're depressed, you tend to eat more, move less, and experience less pleasure in your life.

Although some people lose their appetites when they're depressed, many more overeat in response to feelings of sadness, loneliness, and social isolation. (Depressive eating is a form of emotional eating.) Food temporarily numbs and alleviates negative feelings, and it can even give you a short mood or energy burst. (This is also why some people suffering from depression turn to drugs or alcohol.) But eating because you're depressed will lead only to weight gain and, often, a worsening of depressive symptoms.

Emotional eating isn't the only problem for people with depression. They may also lack the motivation to exercise. The feelings of hopelessness and helplessness can sap your desire to lose weight or get in shape. You may also feel that you just don't have the energy; the lethargy associated with depression can make simply getting out of bed a chore. The sluggishness and fatigue you feel can be a direct side effect of depression, but it may also result from the inability to get a good night's rest, another symptom of depression. And we don't have to tell you just how much exhaustion can affect your eating: When you're feeling tired and drained, you're often not able to make healthy food decisions, even though you *logically* know what they are. As you can see, untreated depression can be a vicious cycle that causes you to pack on extra pounds.

Not surprisingly, a growing body of research suggests that there is an association between obesity and depression. Researchers from the Group Health Cooperative in Seattle found that mood and anxiety disorders, including depression, were about 25 percent more common in obese participants than in their nonobese counterparts. In another study, researchers in the Netherlands found that depressed, overweight individuals had more body image and eating concerns, lower self-esteem, and a higher body mass index (BMI) than nondepressed obese participants. (BMI is a measure of body fat based on height and weight; for more on BMI, turn to appendix 2.) Studies suggest that binge eaters tend to experience depression more frequently than eaters who don't binge. Binge eaters also report that negative moods tend to precede binge episodes, and that their mood is briefly elevated during a binge episode. Depressed people may be at a higher risk of overeating and becoming overweight, especially if food is their main source of pleasure.

Some experts believe that being overweight can increase the risk of depression. It's not easy being overweight in a culture obsessed with thinness, or to live with weight-related stigma and discrimination. Indeed, in a study conducted by Yale University researchers, 35 percent of the respondents said that they would be willing to give up a year of their lives rather than be fat; 30 percent said they would rather be divorced than obese; 25 percent said they would prefer not being able to have children; and 15 percent said they would prefer to be severely depressed. Many obese individuals internalize the prejudice and negative stereotypes, contributing to humiliation, negative body image, low self-esteem, and depression.

Although there is a clear association between being overweight and depression, it's not yet known which is the cause and which is the effect. Researchers don't know whether

A DOCTOR BATTLES DEPRESSION

Michael Foster, a forty-five-year-old physician, sought help to overcome overeating after gaining forty-two pounds in two years. As a physician, he "knew what to do" to lose weight; however, he continued to overeat and reported being too tired to exercise. His mind and best intentions were in conflict with his behaviors.

As the youngest of three boys, Michael grew up in a family dominated by his physician father who worked long hours but spent all of his free time with his wife and kids. Michael's mother struggled with depression and died of breast cancer when he was nine years old. He was close to his father and his brothers, who also became doctors.

After medical school, Michael joined the family-owned medical practice. He lived in the suburbs and enjoyed playing golf and tennis. Nonetheless, he felt trapped in an unhappy marriage and an unfulfilling career. He did not enjoy treating patients full-time, so he decided to pursue his passion for teaching and research. In search of contentment, he divorced his wife, moved to the city, and took a job teaching and conducting research at a medical school. He enjoyed his new work, developed a good rapport with his colleagues, and became well known in his field.

However, in pursuit of tenure, Michael took on more and more professional commitments. He spent ten to twelve hours a day at work, including some weekends. Eventually he felt good only when he was being productive at work. He bought into the Puritan work ethic and became more of a "human doing" than a "human being." He became increasingly weight-related stigma and weight gain due to chronic overeating and physical inactivity lead to depression, or if depression leads to increased appetite, inactivity, weight gain, and negative body image. It's likely that the relationship is symbiotic, if not reciprocal.

Regardless, if depression plays a role in your inability to eat healthfully and exercise regularly, it's important to seek help from a mental health professional in your community who specializes in the treatment of depression. Contact your primary care physician, local mental health center, or your insurance carrier, and ask for names of

isolated on weekends, preferring to stay home, binge on gourmet foods, and drink scotch. Food and alcohol became a distraction, a relief, and a reward.

During his initial assessment, it became clear that Michael was suffering from depression as well as binge eating disorder. Driven to succeed over the past few years, he had become sad and anxious most of the time. Depression had led him to abandon activities like golf and tennis, so that his only pleasures in life were sleeping, eating, and drinking. In retrospect, he realized that as he became increasingly depressed, his appetite and the incidence of overeating had increased.

Michael came to me with a classic case of depression: early loss of a loved one, prolonged periods of sadness and anxiety, loss of interest in usual activities, feelings of hopelessness, difficulty getting up in the morning, and an increased appetite. As I helped him overcome overeating, I also used interpersonal therapy techniques, which address stressful social and interpersonal relationships associated with the onset of depressive symptoms; cognitive behavioral strategies, designed to stop the distorted negative thinking that's linked with depression; and happiness exercises developed by positive psychologists to decrease symptoms of depression.

As Michael's energy increased, he joined a fitness club and resumed playing tennis three times a week. He trained for a bike race sponsored by his hospital. As his depression lifted, he was better able to follow the dietitian's food plans. He became more social, purposefully spending more free time at the health club and seeking out other single adults.

professionals who specialize in depression. If you've resisted the idea of seeking help because you're worried about the potential for weight gain, a side effect of some antidepressant medications, talk to your doctor. She may be able to start you at a lower dosage or use a different medication. And effective nondrug treatments, such as talk therapy and/or stress-relieving strategies, may allow you to use less medication or wean off of it completely.

WHAT CAUSES DEPRESSION?

Many risk factors contribute to depression, including genetics, your biology, and life circumstances. Multiple genes interacting with one another can contribute to depression, and this is passed down from parent to child. So if a family member suffers from depression, your risk is increased. Your biology also can be a factor: Women are much more likely to suffer from depression than men, probably as a result of hormones that affect brain chemistry. Finally, a stressful life event such as a chronic illness, financial stress, or conflicts in a relationship can trigger depression. Past events, too—the early death of a parent or physical, sexual, or emotional abuse—can contribute to depression later in life. Even positive events, like a wedding, a new job, or moving, can be stressful, leaving you feeling exhausted and overwhelmed. Finally, some prescription drugs, such as those used to treat arthritis, heart problems, high cholesterol, high blood pressure, and cancer, can trigger depression. Usually two or more factors are responsible for causing depression.

How can you tell if you're suffering from depression? And could depression be playing a role in your struggle to consistently eat healthfully or robbing you of energy to exercise and engage in other body-positive behaviors? Finding out if you're suffering from depression is the first step to feeling better. If you think you might be depressed, flip to page 236, appendix 3, to take a short survey, called the Goldberg Depression Scale, which will help you identify whether you are, in fact, experiencing symptoms of clinical depression. If your answers reveal that you are suffering from depressive symptoms, the next step is to seek help. Fortunately, there are a number of effective treatments for depression, ranging from talk therapy, to antidepressants, to alternative therapies such as acupuncture and vitamin and mineral supplements. More than 80 percent of people who receive treatment for depression report that it helps them feel better. Seeking treatment will not only improve your mood and outlook on life, but it can also give you the energy and focus to make the changes necessary to lose weight and keep it off.

IDENTIFYING SOURCES OF PAIN

As I've already mentioned in this chapter, you have to pinpoint the cause of your emotional pain before you can get to work on fixing it. For example, if you're angry, ask yourself why are you feeling it now? Do you always try to please others at your own expense because you can't tolerate conflict, and then resent them for taking advantage of your easygoing nature? Whatever your reason, remind yourself that food is not an effective way to deal with stress and pain in your life. Remember, the doughnuts you're eating may taste good now and may make you forget about your alcoholic spouse, but after you finish them, your alcoholic spouse will still be there. And the cycle, unfortunately, will continue: You'll keep turning to food as your spouse keeps turning to the bottle. So now, not only are you dealing with your spouse's drinking problem, you're also dealing with your disordered eating. While emotional eating may serve as a temporary distraction, this self-destructive tactic will persist in creating more problems in your life.

You may have to dig pretty deeply to figure out what's going on, as some of the issues surrounding emotional pain may stem from problems you experienced as a child. For instance, if your needs for love, dependence, or acceptance were not met early in your life, you may have never learned the skills to be in healthy relationships in the present. As a result, you may be at risk of turning to unhealthy alternatives, such as food, drugs, alcohol, overworking, excessive shopping, an Internet addiction, and so forth, to fulfill those needs. You may be overeating because you are unable to engage oth-

WHEN FOOD REPLACES LOVE

Everyone important to Mary Findlay had failed her. Throughout Mary's childhood, her mother became angry whenever Mary needed anything from her because she was exhausted from caring for both Mary's sister, who had cerebral palsy, and her alcoholic husband. The only time her mother would give without resentment was when it related to food and gifts. They ate ice cream sundaes together, and they enjoyed baking cookies together and giving them as presents during the holidays. Mary would go to the candy store to buy pounds of sweets using spare change her father would give her at the end of the week; she'd bring the goodies home to share with her mother and her family. Tragically, at times throughout her childhood, her father came into her room at night when he was drunk and sexually abused her.

Mary learned early in life that people couldn't be counted on and were not safe. But she could always count on food. She overate as a child and continued to overeat as an adult, even though she married a wonderful man who offered her unconditional love and support.

In therapy, Mary realized that for her food was a way to gain nurturance without risking vulnerability. Her obsession with food distracted her from dealing with the disappointment of not feeling loved as a child. Food soothed her when adult friendships didn't last. It kept

ers in gratifying relationships. Spending the night with your favorite companion, Ben and Jerry's, feels safer. Christine Walker, a forty-three-year-old mother of three girls, observes insightfully, "I can turn to food twenty-four hours a day. It never says no. I can depend on it to taste good. It's not going to say, 'You're too needy.'"

Until Mary (see box above) went into therapy, she didn't fully realize that she was using food to soothe traumatic childhood wounds. Sometimes it's not obvious why you're in emotional pain. If you're struggling to find the cause, the exercise below is a good place to start. Write down the specific issues that apply to you under each problem area. If you are an emotional eater, these are some of the core areas in which emotional conflicts can be buried by overeating.

her filled up and safe. In order to change lifelong eating habits, Mary had to take risks and allow herself to be vulnerable with "safe" people like her husband. She also needed to learn the skills necessary to develop healthy relationships, negotiation strategies, and assertiveness techniques. With much courage, she allowed herself to get closer to others and use her newfound relationship enhancement skills. Her need to overeat decreased, and the focus switched from food to people.

However, as Mary lost weight, she became scared and felt vulnerable. She said, "I thought I would love losing weight and look forward to buying beautiful new clothes. But I don't; I feel scared. When I go to the mall, men smile at me, and I'm afraid they will follow me out to my car. In the past, because I felt fat and big, when my tall husband hugged me, I never felt vulnerable. Now I feel small and insecure in his embrace, as if I will be taken advantage of or hurt."

It took time for Mary to realize that she was no longer the young girl who couldn't escape abusive experiences at the hands of her parents. She learned to feel and act like a confident adult, trusting that her husband was not going to take advantage of her because she was "smaller." She grew to know that if men approached her, she would be able to protect herself through assertive words and actions.

MAJOR PROBLEM AREAS

1. Family conflicts (current or past)

2. Work and school conflicts

3. Toxic relationships

4. Money worries

5. Health issues (including an unhealthy lifestyle)

6. Unresolved loss/grief

DIFFERENTIATING HEALTHY RELATIONSHIPS FROM TOXIC ONES

Many—sometimes all—of the major problem areas listed on the previous page stem from relationships. In some cases, it's obvious that a relationship is the issue: For instance, a family conflict or a toxic relationship very clearly involves our interactions with others. But work conflicts and other job-related issues may also be caused by relationship problems, such as not getting along with your boss or a coworker. Your money worries, too, could have a relationship issue at their core. Perhaps your spouse spends too much money, or shopping fills the same role for you as food, helping you cope with relationship issues. An unhealthy lifestyle could also reflect the way that you deal with people: Maybe you pour all your energies into others and don't take enough time for yourself. It's even possible that the relationship issue you struggle with may not involve anyone else at all—it could be a result of your relationship with yourself. Then again, some of these problems may not be connected to anyone else, but because relationships can be such a major source of unhappiness, you should give yourself some time to thoroughly explore them.

As you do so, I'd like you to pay special attention to the relationship you have with your parents, because this can give you a lot of insight into your emotional eating. We often learn to love and take care of ourselves from the way we were loved and taken care of as children by our parents. In most cultures, females are primarily responsible for the nurturing role. Mothers are usually the ones who feed us; clothe us; and provide attention, affection, support, and guidance, so your relationship with your mother can be very telling. (As women have become an even greater part of the workforce, fathers are increasingly becoming more involved in the act of parenting their children, so you may have to also explore your relationship with your father to learn more about your issues with others and food.)

What happens, then, when you grow up with a mother who is emotionally damaged and is extremely needy herself? What are the effects of being raised by a mom who is depressed, overwhelmed, deprived, and even angry about having to respond to the natural needs of a child? When a woman is unable to mother her child, oftentimes the roles switch and the child becomes the parent. You may have learned to ignore or distract yourself from your own needs and become focused on fulfilling everyone else's needs. You probably became self-sufficient at an early age, doing things for yourself that most other kids' mothers did for them. You may have become overly sensitive and driven to meet your mother's needs and to make her happy.

That caretaker or mother role that you assumed isn't limited to that particular parent-child relationship—it can also spill over into your friendships, your marriage, and your relationships with your children and even your coworkers. Because you're an expert at anticipating and taking care of others' needs, you probably gravitate toward needy people. That's what you're used to. You are comfortable in this role and become the selfless mother, ever-giving husband, or overly dedicated friend. You remain unaware of your own suppressed neediness because you focus on the needs of others.

But over the years, this driven and relentless giving to others of what you never received yourself becomes more and more frustrating and exhausting. The result is that you increasingly feel deprived, resentful, and hungry all the time. You may finish breakfast and then obsess about what you will eat for lunch all morning. It keeps you distracted and out of touch with any yearnings of your own for attention, care, and respect. You may live with chronic dissatisfaction from being trapped in unsatisfactory relationships in which you give a lot and get little back. When feelings of resentment, loneliness, or exhaustion enter your consciousness, you head to the kitchen to eat.

If this is your situation, then you've been hungry a long time—hungry for the comfort of a warm, nurturing voice, loving touch, and wisdom and guidance from another. It's time to become conscious of the hungers and needs that you have disowned and locked away to survive childhood. You now have to learn to listen to your body, to acknowledge your profound hunger for the mothering that your mother was not able to give. Try sitting with these newly conscious and intense hungers, share them with others, or even keep a journal about them. Then make a commitment to nurture and mother yourself.

Ultimately, you should take some time to assess *all* of your relationships—including the one you have with yourself—to see if they play a role in your struggle with emotional eating. You may notice a trend or a vicious cycle in which the same people and situations can trigger repetitive emotional eating. To help you understand how your relationships lead to emotional overeating, ask yourself four questions:

1. Who are the three people I am closest to?

   Examples: Your work colleague, your sister, and your best friend from childhood.

2. How do I eat before, while, and after I am with them? Is there a pattern?

   Example: On Monday mornings before work, you always meet your colleague to "start off the work week." You notice that you eat two bagels instead of one and that you're scarfing down your food.

3. What are my expectations of them?

   Example: I want my colleague to complete her own work and not expect me to cover for her when she overextends her lunch hour or wants to leave early. I want her to listen to me when we meet on Mondays rather than the whole conversation focusing on her.

4. What can I do to help me feel better when these people don't meet my expectations without straying from my weight loss or healthy lifestyle plan? (It's important to realize that no one can be there for you 24/7. You have to have other sources of fuel and comfort available. Later in this chapter, we will talk about finding healthier alternatives to food.)

Example: Rather than hoping that your colleague will just do the right thing or read your mind, tell her you're uncomfortable covering for her and that she needs to find another way to manage her time and work demands. And discuss sharing time at your Monday breakfasts.

BARRIER: STRESS FROM BEING OVEREXTENDED AND OVERSCHEDULED

The questions and demands start from the moment you wake up. Do the kids have to be picked up after school? Did I write up the summary of the PTA meeting? What should I wear? When will I visit my mother in the nursing home? Which email should I return first? Should I be answering my cell phone or my home phone? What will we have for dinner tonight?

BREATHING: AN INSTANT STRESS BREAKER

Need a simple way to soothe stress? Just breathe. Breathing, which is something you can easily control and regulate, can help you feel more relaxed and clear your mind. Whenever you feel frazzled or tense, try taking five to ten minutes to practice the following breathing exercise. Feel free to repeat it several times a day.

Start by finding a quiet, comfortable space where you will not be interrupted. Sit with your back straight, close your eyes, and quietly inhale through your nose, and say to yourself, *Rising*, as your chest rises. Then exhale completely through your mouth to the count of six and say to yourself, *Falling,* as your chest falls. Your mind will wander, and when it does, simply label the thought and then return to taking a deep breath: *Rising.* So if you think about a project at work, simply say to yourself, *Work,* then return to your breath.

Deep breathing is one of the best ways to lower stress because it sends a message to the brain to calm down and relax. Your brain, in turn, sends a message to your body to slow your heart rate, lower blood pressure, and unwind.

When the demands in your life outnumber the resources, your stress level skyrockets. Even if you can keep this juggling act going, at least one person is going to suffer: you! To cope with the excessive demands of life, you turn to food. How did things get to this point? Often, it's that you're a giving person—too giving—and you need more boundaries. You have a hard time saying no. There are lots of reasons for that, including the desire for approval, the need to feel indispensable, the feeling that people won't like or love you unless you do—actually, *over*do—for them. You might not consider yourself worthy of getting your own needs met.

LIBERATED BY A NEW JOB DESCRIPTION

Susan Bronell, a forty-five-year-old mother of twin college freshman, sought therapy to stop bingeing and lose weight permanently. When the twins were in high school, she worked part-time as a nurse and was active in the PTA and her kids' sports organizations. She was an incredible mother who had a hard time saying no, and as a result, she struggled with emotional eating for ten years.

In the fall, the boys went away to college; Susan decided it was time to work on herself. She took a cooking class, started exercising regularly, and participated in a twenty-week therapy group for overeaters. She did amazingly well, stopped overeating, and began to train for a fitness event that kept her active for months.

She had more time for herself because she was no longer burdened with cooking, cleaning, and looking after her children. She and her husband enjoyed a more relaxed lifestyle; they went out to eat twice a week. Some nights they kept it simple at home, enjoying a glass of wine, cheese, bread, salad, and fruit. Although she loved being a mom, she embraced the freedom of not having children at home.

When the boys returned from college in May, they dropped their dirty clothes in the laundry room and said they hated the dorm food and couldn't wait to eat some home-cooked meals. Mary was excited to see them, but not to cook their nightly dinners, launder their clothes, and pick up after them again. When she begrudgingly resumed these caretaking habits, she began overeating again.

Most people are able to drop some weight once they start dieting, but if you haven't dealt with the fact that you're constantly overscheduled and exhausted, you will eventually overeat again; the weight loss won't last. Until you can say no to others, you won't be able to say no to food.

Emotional eating is both a reaction to poor boundaries—you eat because you're so stressed out from doing so much for others—and, in itself, a loss of boundaries. When you are eating healthfully, you enjoy the smell, texture, and taste of food, and then you are done. You may brush your teeth or move to another part of the house for the rest of

She returned to therapy for a "booster" session and to get back on track with healthy eating. She shared that she loved her sons, but she had gotten used to the freedom she'd gained while they were away. Mary said she was resentful that they did their own laundry for nine months at college but wanted her to do it now.

Once again, she needed to be reminded that she couldn't consistently set boundaries with food until she consistently set them in other areas of her life. Her job description as a mother to twin eight-year-old boys was different than that for two nineteen-year-old men. Susan needed to update her job description. She had to ask herself: *What do I still need to do for them, and what do they need to do for themselves?*

She decided that it was no longer her job to do their laundry or to cook nightly dinners. She told her sons that she would cook three nights during the week, the family would share carry-out food one night, and on Friday, Saturday, and Sunday they would be on their own. She also let them know that since they'd done their laundry all year at school, they would need to do it for themselves at home as well.

Soon Susan found that she enjoyed her time with her sons more and felt less burdened by others' demands. She was back to eating healthfully and exercising, and she lost the weight she had regained. Setting better boundaries gave her more room to enjoy both her relationships with food and with people.

the night and enjoy your evening activities. But if after dinner you eat the food left on your kids' plates and then go to the freezer for ice cream, you are experiencing a loss of boundaries. The meal is over, and you should be done. Make sure that you fill your plate with enough healthy foods to leave you satisfied. If you do and you're still eating, that's a problem. Lacking boundaries leaves you lacking: You can't consistently set boundaries with food until you set them in other areas of your life. Once you're able to establish some healthy boundaries in your life, you'll find that you're not as overscheduled, stressed, or chaotic, which can help reduce emotional eating. You'll be more relaxed and have the focus and energy to do what is needed for long-term weight loss.

So how do you go about setting boundaries? I recommend creating a job description for yourself as Susan did (page 66). Many companies give out a job description—basically a list of work responsibilities—to new employees. Drawing up a job description for your life can be just as useful; once you outline your responsibilities in life, it's easier to set boundaries for yourself and others.

As you write your job description, take some time to think about who and what you're responsible for in your life: Is it just you? Your spouse? Your children? Your parents? Think about what's realistic in terms of caring for yourself and these other people in your life. Should you be in charge of all household tasks—cooking, cleaning, laundry, and so on—or should these be shared? Are there some tasks that you can delegate to others, including family members, friends, and coworkers? Part of setting appropriate boundaries is learning which responsibilities in your life you can let go of and who can take them on.

BALANCE YOUR DEMANDS AND RESOURCES

We're all trying to find a balance between the demands in our lives and the resources we have to deal with them. When you know which foods you should be eating but can't seem to do it, it's often a sign you need to increase your resources or decrease your demands. You'll need to pay attention to what's going on in your life, sometimes on a day-to-day basis, to make sure there's a balance between the two. To get a clear picture, use the following worksheet.

Start by writing down your demands, or all the tasks you need to do in a given day, in the left column. It might include things like taking your children to school, going food shopping, getting to work, and so on. In the right-hand column, list the resources you have to deal with those demands. Resources are concrete sources of help, such as a neighbor who can drop your child off at school or an inheritance a family member has left you that you can put toward a babysitter or bills. Resources also include enjoyable activities that help reduce tension. Time with friends, exercise, meditation, involvement in a spiritual community such as your church, Overeaters Anonymous, or even an on-line support group are all resources.

DEMANDS VERSUS RESOURCES

Demands	*Resources*

Take a look at what you've written. Is the Demands column longer than the Resources column? Are you working too many hours? Do you have too many responsibilities? When stressful demands outnumber resources, symptoms like overeating or drinking arise in response to the pain or discomfort of an unbalanced lifestyle. To keep these symptoms from worsening or to prevent them altogether, change is required—whether that entails giving up certain things in your life, delegating them to others, or asking for more help or support from friends or family members. If you don't do this, you will continue to engage in unhealthy behaviors in an attempt to numb the pain of living this way. Another great exercise that can help restore balance in your life is Bob's Circle of Life, which you can find on his website, www.thebestlife.com.

BARRIER: INABILITY TO DELAY GRATIFICATION

For long-term weight loss to occur, you have to develop the capacity to delay gratification, and this involves strengthening your willpower. Emotional eaters typically want to feel good fast. For example, if you're an emotional eater and you're upset about a fight you had with a family member, a bowl of ice cream or a handful of cookies will take the edge off in just a few minutes. True, it's a temporary fix, but it's a fix nonetheless. People who use healthy coping techniques, however, don't necessarily get this relief right away. Instead of turning to food, they might sit and think about the argument, come up with some solutions or compromises, and then call the family member to discuss the problem. After some initial discomfort, the person is able to resolve the problem. As you can see, the latter technique involves insight and emotional strength.

Fortunately, researchers have found that we can increase willpower. It's like a muscle; the more we use it, the stronger it gets. Taking time to appreciate the things you value in life, thinking positively or even laughing, can help you build your resolve. Another way to develop willpower: Practice postponing gratification. The following exercise can help you do just that.

LEARNING TO WAIT

When you go into the kitchen hunting around for food, ask yourself this: Are you really physically hungry, or are you bored, thirsty, lonely, and so on? (You can use the Hunger Scale on pages 230–231 to assess this.) If the answer is "I just ate dinner, so I'm not

THE BREAKDOWN OF A BINGE

You were going to have just one cookie, and you had five—is that a binge? Maybe, maybe not. Or perhaps you went back into the kitchen after dinner and polished off a package of cheese, six frozen waffles, a half jar of peanut butter, and a pint of ice cream, all the while feeling powerless to stop. Now, *that's* definitely a binge. While the term is used loosely to describe overeating, for psychologists, nutritionists, and others who deal with eating issues, bingeing involves two factors: eating a large quantity of food and feeling out of control. So the occasional overeating to the tune of five medium-sized cookies, with no negative impact on your life, probably isn't a binge. But if you felt very out of control eating those cookies, well, then you're starting to get into binge territory.

Along with anorexia (pathological undereating) and bulimia (bingeing and purging), psychologists are giving serious consideration to officially creating a separate and distinct eating disorder called binge eating disorder. This involves bingeing that is *not* followed by self-induced vomiting, as in bulimia. Recent research suggests that the disorder is more common than anorexia and bulimia. One study sponsored by the National Institute of Mental Health indicates that about 3.5 percent of women and 2 percent of men have had binge eating disorders in their lifetime, making it four times as prevalent as anorexia and about twice as common as bulimia.

Bingeing, in the clinical sense, is an extreme form of using food to cope. Bingers describe the feeling as numbing and exhilarating but at the same time shameful and painful (emotionally and literally, as the stomach stretches to accommodate all that food). If you're a binger, many of the issues you're addressing in this chapter and in the next chapter—eliminating major sources of stress, learning new coping skills, changing your taste preferences—can help resolve your bingeing problem.

hungry," wait fifteen minutes. Say to yourself, *I can eat all I want then, but first I have to wait it out.*

During the fifteen-minute wait, do whatever you want except eat. Read a magazine, check your email, listen to your favorite music, or write in your journal. You may also want to use the time to figure out why you want to eat. Perhaps it's because you don't feel like doing something else you're supposed to do, like write thank-you cards or work on taxes. It's important to understand what behavior or emotion you're avoiding when you turn to food for gratification. Make a mental list of what's still on your to-do list that may be stressing or "eating at" you. Then ask yourself, *Will eating now add to or subtract from these pressures or demands? What behavior* will *help me reduce my tension?*

After fifteen minutes, you may decide that you don't need the food, which is ideal. If you do decide to eat, or even to binge, place the food(s) and the amounts you typically eat, if you can recall from previous overeating or bingeing episodes, on a counter or table. Why do this? Because it forces you to ask: *How many ice-cream sandwiches might I eat? How much cheese and crackers? How many chips?* And so forth. When you see all that food in front of you, you may be surprised. You may find yourself thinking instead, *I'll have just one ice-cream sandwich or two handfuls of chips.* This exercise helps you to slow down the process of overeating and develop the capacity to delay gratification and self-regulate.

HANDLING FEELINGS WITHOUT FOOD

After reading through the common barriers to overcoming emotional eating, you may have had a few realizations. Even if there were no surprises, perhaps you got confirmation that, yes, this is your issue and you now understand it better. By figuring out why you use food to cope with emotions and why you've struggled to stop, you can now take steps to fix it. That's what this next exercise is about.

Step 1: Question Yourself

The next time you feel like mainlining a pizza, stop and ask yourself the following questions:

1. Am I really physically hungry?

2. What emotional state am I experiencing now? Label it. (Example: "I am sad because my sister was just diagnosed with breast cancer.")

3. Decide how to handle your feelings. (Example: Call her. Empathize with her. Offer help. Talk to your husband and tell him: "I would like to go to California to help my sister during her treatments.")

4. Learn to tolerate the reactions of others. (Example: In an ideal world, everyone would be understanding of the fact that you want to help your sister, but unfortunately, that's not always the case. If your husband responds negatively to your decision—perhaps he gives you a hard time about going and complains about having to take care of the kids while you're away—try to hear him out without being defensive. Let him know that you understand and respect the dilemma this will impose, but this is something you have to do.)

5. Be assertive. Clearly, calmly, and confidently tell others what you plan to do to address their concerns. (Example: You will help make arrangements for someone to take care of the kids for two weekends while you're away.)

6. Accept the responses of others. (Example: Your husband may still be unhappy, saying that you shouldn't be putting your sister's needs before your family's. But applaud yourself for doing what's right for you and your sister. Explain to your husband that it's important that you be there to help your sister during this difficult time—not just for her but for you. Explain that you'll do all you can to make

your absence as easy as it can be for him and the kids. At this point, take a moment to remind yourself that you don't need to give in to the stress or feelings of guilt and binge: "I need to be strong and speak up for myself.")

Answering these questions can be discomforting, even painful, but it's critical. If you don't take the time to ask them and be honest with yourself, you'll miss a golden opportunity to not only fend off overeating or an all-out binge but also gain a sense of control over your eating and yourself. When emotions run high—emotions that you may bury the rest of the day; emotions that are the very reason you overeat—you become vulnerable to an overeating episode. The above questions will help you identify these emotions and label them, which helps make them easier to handle.

Step 2: Find a Healthy Replacement

Whenever you want to cuddle up with your favorite security blanket—food—reach for a healthier coping tool. It can be an object (for instance, a T-shirt that makes you feel comfortable and safe), a person (such as a friend who can lift your mood), an activity (like going for a walk or run, or watching a movie), or something spiritual (a prayer that gives you perspective). In fact, you might want to make a list of all the things that help relax, soothe, and comfort you or provide entertainment and stimulation. Learning how to shift moods with music, movies, exercise, books, and prayer *instead of food* is crucial for long-term weight loss success.

To figure out what healthy coping tools you should use, review the following list. Then you can turn to these things when you're otherwise tempted to turn to eating. It might not always work, especially at first, but in time it will help you gradually change your thinking and reactions. Remember, a little bit of change each day leads to major change over time. When the urge to overeat strikes, instead focus on:

1. **Music:** Does classical, folk, jazz, Christian, new age, country, or rock help you shift moods or feel energized or relaxed when you need it? Put CDs of this type of music on your list.

2. **Movies:** What movies help you change moods? Dramas? Comedies? Romances? Musicals? Action films? Jot down the names of the DVDs that soothe your soul or get you moving.

3. **Clothes:** Do you prefer sweats, warm pj's, old sweaters from someone you love, or warm, fluffy blankets? Does that vibrant yellow T-shirt brighten your mood? What clothes, colors, and fabrics make you feel comfortable and safe? Use your list to keep an inventory of these clothes, and pull them out when you feel cold, empty, or lonely.

4. **Exercise:** Does taking a walk calm you down? Or maybe going for a bike ride or pedaling your exercise bike in the basement while watching TV? Exercise is a fantastic stress reliever, and, as you'll read in chapter 4, also a mood booster. Exercise is also an extremely effective way to deal with the emotional pain that I mentioned earlier. This might seem like a contradiction; many people avoid exercise because it's painful or uncomfortable. But, interestingly, exercise actually increases our tolerance to both physical and emotional pain. In a way, we can become almost bulletproof as we increase our strength and endurance. Your perspective changes after you've experienced the discipline of training, especially if you trained for a race and crossed the finish line. You might think, *What's the big deal of simply confronting someone when I've pounded out all those miles?* (For more on exercise and where to start, check out appendix 6, starting on page 255.) So make a note of the activities you find most satisfying and relaxing.

5. **Family and friends:** With whom do you enjoy spending time? Jot down the names of these people. Bonding with family members, catching up with friends, meeting new people, or getting to know people in your neighborhood serves a dual pur-

pose: Not only do they fill up your time, leaving you less time to overeat, but they also help fulfill you. We're often hesitant to reach out to friends or family members—people are so busy. But a support system of people who encourage your new healthy lifestyle is critical to staying balanced and motivated. And remember, you can offer people as much as or more than you take. So pick up the phone, chat, make plans to go out. And if texting or emailing does the trick and keeps you away from the chips and cookies, then go for it! Refer back to the "Demands versus Resources" list you drew up: Are there enough people in your resource list to offer you support? If not, work on establishing new friendships. And consider a support group, either in person or online. Mary Jo Schneider, profiled in chapter 1, credits Overeaters Anonymous for her weight maintenance success.

6. **Crafts:** What forms of creative expression do you enjoy? Add these to your list. Knitting a sweater for your grandchild, sculpting clay to express your feelings, creating homemade cards for those you love, putting together a scrapbook of happy memories or good times—all of these are ways to positively distract or enliven yourself, or channel your negative thoughts and feelings.

7. **Unmet goals:** What's the one thing you've always wanted to do? Have you dreamed of scuba diving or jumping out of an airplane? Do you want to learn a new language or backpack through Europe? Put these on your list, and when you're tempted to use food to cope, instead take some time to map out how to make these dreams a reality. You'll find it infinitely more rewarding and enjoyable than overeating.

8. **Spirituality:** Which prayers, inspirational books, sacred objects (such as a rosary or a bell for meditation) inspire you during times when you want to give in and binge or overeat? Make a note of the spiritual symbols or books that you can reach for when you want to reach for food.

9. **Charity work:** What are some nonprofit groups or organizations with which you'd like to work? By volunteering at a soup kitchen, helping out at a church clothing

drive, or working on raising funds for a community center, you get the joy of helping others in need—an obvious perk. Plus, you're able to bond with other people as you work toward a common goal, which can also make you feel good about yourself.

10. **Community:** How can you get involved in your neighborhood? Whether you take a class or seminar at your local high school, attend civic or school board meetings, or become an EMT, you'll feel invested in your community, which can help give your life meaning and purpose. Look through your local newspaper to find events and meetings that spark your interest.

11. What else can you add to your list that can replace food as a way to deal with uncomfortable feelings, people, or situations? _____

_____

_____

_____

ACHIEVE YOUR GOALS

I've given you a lot to think about and a lot of strategies to try. Where to begin? Start with one specific goal that you can work on today, tomorrow, or sometime this week at the latest to overcome emotional eating. To close in on your goal, think back to which of the exercises in this chapter most resonated with you. Perhaps you want to try waiting fifteen minutes before eating. Or maybe you want to work on setting boundaries by drawing up a job description. Here are a couple of examples of goals you can set; feel free to come up with your own or tweak these.

1. **Add a new resource.** If in completing the exercise on page 69, you find you're short on resources, use the goal-setting worksheet on the following page to plan how you're going to find extra resources. For example, "I'll do my grocery shopping online each week and have the packages delivered to the house. That way, I can use

the time I would have spent at the store to go to the gym." Or, "On Saturdays, I'll take the baby to my mother-in-law's for three hours so I can prepare a few healthy meals for the week."

2. **Find nonfood ways to relax.** If you discover in the Lifestyle Log that you turn to food to cope with stress, then look at the list of suggestions beginning on page 75, or come up with other ways to soothe and comfort yourself. For instance, you could plan to keep snacks out of your desk drawer and take a fifteen-minute walk during your lunch break. Or schedule a night out with your spouse or a friend once a week.

Setting a goal is only the first step—you also have to devise a plan to achieve it. That's where the goal-setting worksheet comes into play. It can help you map out a timeline, pinpoint potential barriers, and create strategies to overcome them. Check out the sample worksheet below for inspiration, then turn to appendix 4 to begin your own. (You can also download copies for free at www.thebestlife.com/motivation.) After you set your goal, check back in with your worksheet after twenty-four hours to make sure everything is going smoothly. If you need to make any adjustments, do so then. Give yourself two weeks to work on your chosen goal. Hopefully, by then you should be in the routine of doing it, and it will become a good habit. After the two weeks are up, set a new two-week goal, and so on.

WHAT YOUR GOAL-SETTING WORKSHEET MIGHT LOOK LIKE

1. **What is my emotional-eating goal?** Choose a realistic goal you feel you can achieve. For example: "I want to cut down my episodes of overeating at night."

2. **What is the most positive outcome of achieving this goal?** It's important that you can identify the advantages of working toward your goal; this will serve as powerful motivation. For instance: "I won't feel so helpless, out of control, and disgusted with myself after I pig out. Plus, not eating so many calories at night would certainly help me lose weight."

3. **What is the main obstacle standing in my way?** For example: "I have overeaten at night ever since I was in college, and I'm afraid that if I stop doing so, I will not be able to calm down and unwind enough to get to sleep."

4. **How can I overcome the obstacle?** Give specifics, such as how you'll do it and when. For example: "I'll develop a new routine that helps me settle down at the end of the day. After dinner, I can walk my dog and play with the kids, then read a book for a while after they go to bed. Before I go to bed, I can play soft, relaxing music and practice deep breathing exercises."

5. **How do I prevent the obstacle from occurring in the first place?** Again, focus on how and when. For instance: "I may have to lessen my demands so that I am not so wound up at the end of the day. I could put my kids in bed earlier so that I have some downtime to relax before bed."

6. **How, specifically, should I achieve my emotional-eating goal?** Be as specific as possible, focusing once more on how and when. For example: "I can have dinner with the kids at six o'clock, then clean up the kitchen and enjoy the kids. I will put them to bed at eight instead of nine-thirty, and between eight and ten o'clock, I can engage in relaxing, enjoyable activities to replace binge eating."

In this chapter, I've outlined a bunch of strategies to help you recognize and overcome emotional eating once and for all. You've learned how to tolerate feelings, and accept and learn from them so that you no longer have to numb them or stuff them down with food. You've learned techniques to set boundaries and change your relationships with others, and you've also learned how to get *your* needs met through people instead of food. You've learned strategies for strengthening your willpower and delaying gratification. Remember, developing a healthy relationship with food is a process, so I encourage you to check back into this chapter whenever you need a refresher or a motivation boost.

3

REWIRING YOUR SUGAR-, FAT-, AND SALT-LOVING BRAIN

By Janis Jibrin

WE'VE ALL GOTTEN UP from a table feeling way too stuffed, or told ourselves we'd have just one cookie, but then had another, and then a few more. Very few people have perfect control around food, and, fortunately, your body can deal with occasional lapses. But when overeating becomes the norm, and you're out of control around food, it can be bewildering. What's happening is that a very real, very powerful set of forces—from your physiological makeup to the environment you live in—are driving you to overdo it. Understanding those forces, and how to outsmart them, is what this chapter is all about.

Feeling controlled by food isn't easy to admit to yourself, much less to others. I had a client, whom I'll call Carol, who for months faithfully showed up at my office every Thursday. We'd pore over her food record, searching for clues as to why this highly accomplished lawyer, mother, and wife was one hundred pounds too heavy. High-fiber cereal for breakfast, equally nutritious foods for lunch and dinner, the occasional controlled splurge—it all looked so good. Obviously, it was *too* good. She lost a few pounds and then told me she was too busy to come back. A year later, I got an email from her confessing that she was a food addict who sneaked candy, cookies, and chips when no one was looking. She wrote, "Like any good addict, I lied about what I was doing because I was embarrassed. Without my being honest, there really wasn't a way for you to help me. I had to get desperate enough. Eventually, it became more painful to carry on as I was than it was to admit my addiction." When Carol started working on her food addiction—using many of the techniques you'll find in this chapter—weight loss was a natural side effect. She's been at a healthy weight for two and half years, and maintaining gets easier all the time.

Carol may have been able to own up to and deal with her food addiction sooner if she'd known that it's largely not her fault. If you struggle with your eating, I'm hoping that learning about all the forces that drive you to overeat will help you let go of some of the shame and guilt that come from being controlled by food—emotions that only interfere with your efforts to trim down.

The thing to remember is that while the drive to overeat is strong, you're more powerful. It may not seem this way when you're face to face with a double chocolate cake or you're staring down a platter of French fries, but it's true. You just need to find the right techniques that will put you back in control of your eating, your weight, and, ultimately, your health and happiness. And no diet can do this for you. In fact, going on a diet may be the worst thing you can do. Instead, you need to arm yourself with new ways of relating to food, thinking about food, and, incidentally, *not* thinking about food. I'll share my full arsenal with you in this chapter. But first I'll explain the forces that compel you to overeat and keep you overweight, despite your best efforts.

As we work together throughout this chapter, I want you to know that I get it—I know how hard it is to break bad habits and form new ones. As a sweets lover, I've struggled for years. I can tell you what's in every bakery within a five-mile radius of my home, and I'm on a first-name basis with the people who run Biagio Fine Chocolate, located just around the corner. Fortunately, I can now enjoy sweets without being controlled by them, because I'm using the same strategies I'll be recommending to you. So now I'm in control of *when* I go to these places, and *what* I walk out with.

WHAT KIND OF EATER ARE YOU?

Among people who overeat, I typically see three different types: garden-variety over-eater, food abuser, and, like my client Carol, food addict. Any of these three types may also be an emotional eater, which makes converting to a healthy way of eating even more challenging—but still doable.

Garden-variety overeaters are the least controlled by food; they're not obsessing over it all the time, and they may not even experience strong cravings. Perhaps the reason they overeat is because they grew up eating big portions at home and/or often eat out in restaurants, where they clean their plate (generally featuring an oversized portion) without much thought. Or they might not eat big portions, but out of habit or lack of nutrition knowledge, they make really fattening choices (steaks, fries, soft drinks), so they wind up taking in too many calories. Or their overeating might be caused by emotions, as Ann covered in the previous chapter.

Food abusers are more under the grip of food. Like drug and alcohol abusers, they do experience cravings and often give in to them even though their habit causes serious problems in their lives: like being overweight and the spin-off social and health consequences.

Food addicts not only abuse food but also experience the same things that people with drug and alcohol addictions do: They need more of the substance to achieve the same effect, and they experience withdrawal symptoms. While anyone who's ever felt controlled by a chocolate chip cookie has no doubt that he or she is addicted, the terms "food addict" and "addictive food" are still somewhat controversial in the scientific community. Food addiction is not an official condition recognized by the medical field, but more and more researchers agree that it's a real diagnosis.

No matter what type of eater you are—addict, abuser, or garden-variety over-eater—the nine step treatment plan starting on page 98 will help break the spell that food holds over you.

WHY DO YOU OVEREAT?

So, why is the bowl of M&M's sitting on the conference room table so distracting that you can't concentrate on the meeting until you grab a handful? Why do you order dessert when you're still stuffed from dinner? Why do you do things like open a box of minidoughnuts on your way back from the supermarket, swearing you'll eat just one, and then end up polishing off the entire box by the time you pull into your driveway? Why do cravings always seem to get the better of you? Whether you're a garden-variety overeater, a food abuser, or a food addict, your overeating problem is not simply a lack of willpower. Below are some of the primary reasons why, despite what you may want to do (eat healthfully, avoid sweets, lose weight, and so on), you still struggle to actually do it. In other words, these are the barriers to eating a healthy, balanced diet that you'll need to overcome or find a way to deal with if you want to get your eating and your weight back under control. (That's what we'll be working on in the Nine Step Program.)

YOU INHERITED A CAVEMAN'S BRAIN

Go back about one hundred thousand years to the time when cavemen roamed the earth (the Paleolithic Age, in case you're wondering). That's when many of our food preferences were established. Because pulling together a meal took real effort—in the form of hunting and gathering—human survival was determined by a person's ability to seek out foods that were safe (not toxic), nutritious, and high in calories. That's how our tastes for sweet, fatty, salty (a little sodium is necessary for survival), and high-protein (savory) foods evolved. It's also how our ability to perceive bitter taste, which warned us away from potentially poisonous foods, and sour taste, signaling "proceed with caution," developed.

Plus, we were attracted to variety. New tastes and flavors—even just the anticipation of them—spark our brain's pleasure centers. Again, this was all about survival: The more types of plant and animal foods our ancestors ate, the more likely that they would cover their vitamin and mineral needs. Then on top of all of this, a different set of hormones evolved to make sure that people packed on fat, in case they ever had to draw from their reserves. All of this made perfect sense in a time when calories were hard won.

But it clearly makes no sense in a world where all you have to do to indulge your taste for fat and salt is get in your car and pick up a 1,000-plus-calorie meal at the drive-thru. Or where your urge for variety takes you to Baskin-Robbins, where, over the years, more than one thousand different flavors of ice cream have been created. This drive for variety is also the reason why no matter how full you feel after a meal, you suddenly have room for dessert. No problem if you were eating a caveman's dessert—a 40-calorie handful of berries—but with our built-in penchant for fat and sweets, it's pretty difficult to resist the hundreds of calories in cookies, cakes, pies, and sundaes.

But the good news: You can retrain your tastes and actually get to the point where you enjoy—even prefer—healthier foods. (It's true!) And you can rein in the instinct for variety and actually use it to your advantage.

YOUR BRAIN GETS STUCK ON THE BAD HABITS YOU'VE CREATED

Whenever you repeatedly give in to high-fat, indulgent foods, you create a habit. For instance, if you always eat in front of the TV or when you go to the mall, or if you typically eat at a certain time (your two o'clock trek to the vending machine) or with a specific person (your reliable binge buddy), you're conditioning yourself to expect food in these situations. It carves a pathway into the brain, and the more you repeat the behavior, the deeper the groove in the brain becomes. And if eating the food temporarily quells stress, loneliness, or other emotions, now emotions have become another trigger (as you've read about in chapter 2). The next time you're stressed out or in emotional pain, your brain seeks out those foods again, which once more brings temporary relief. With each turn of the cycle, the connection between food and mood gets stronger and more reinforced in the brain.

You can unlink addictive foods from their triggers. I'm not saying that breaking these types of habits is easy, but you can do it and still have a life full of pleasure. In fact, you'll have even more pleasure. After all, our hardwired tastes for food aren't the only source of gratification. Feeling in control of your life as well as the sense of pride and accomplishment—and relief—that you broke a destructive habit also tickle the pleasure centers of the brain in a big way. Which, in turn, only helps further ingrain your new healthier habits.

YOUR BRAIN GETS A HIGH OFF FOOD

You may not be exaggerating when you say you're "addicted" to a food or that you get a "high" after eating your favorite sweet. In fact, the way the brain responds to addictive foods can be strikingly similar to its response to drugs or alcohol. For instance, some of the brain chemicals, such as opioids and endocannabinoids, that are released by eating certain foods, are, as they sound, the body's own version of opium and cannabis (marijuana), and they share the same brain receptors as these drugs. A receptor is like a lock located either on a cell's surface or inside a cell; it takes a specific "key" (for instance an opioid) to fit into the lock and trigger a reaction. (Most likely, you've already heard of endorphins, which are the best-known type of opioids.) These "feel-good" brain chemicals have one job in common: to keep you coming back for more tasty, high-calorie foods, a trait that was so critical for our caveman ancestors' survival.

And, of course, the foods that give us the biggest spike in feel-good chemicals aren't apples or whole grains. "The brain chemical rush from doughnuts, hot dogs, or other high-fat and/or high-sugar foods is so strong that you keep going back for another rush," says Stephanie Fulton, PhD, a professor at the Faculty of Medicine, University of Montreal in Canada, who researches food and brain-reward circuitry.

This brain chemical rush is only partly responsible for the drive to eat, though. A number of other things occur in the body, all of which get you primed to eat: Your thoughts turn to food, your sense of smell becomes sharper, and you actually get spurred on to seek out food. One study showed that when people were injected with the appetite-stimulating hormone ghrelin, not only did their appetite increase, but they started vividly imagining and describing their favorite meal. And another hormone, orexin, both stimulates our muscles to move when we're hungry and strengthens our sense of smell, which made it easier for our ancestors to find food.

YOUR WIRING MAY BE A LITTLE OFF

If what I've just described above sounds hard enough to contend with, imagine having an amped-up version of this wiring. Believe it or not, some people are even more vulnerable to food, the smells and the pleasure hit that eating brings, because the brain wiring that makes them turn to fatty, sweet, and salty foods is "supercharged." Compared to others, they get even more of an opioid rush from food, which drives them to keep going back for more.

Up until only recently, researchers had to rely on what people said about the pleasure they derived from eating to support this theory. For instance, men and women who score higher on questionnaires that indicate what researchers call "reward sensitivity"—the amount of pleasure and sense of reward that people say they get from food—tend to eat a lot more junk food and be more overweight. In a Canadian study, the subjects who scored highest in reward sensitivity tests were 50 percent more likely to be frequent visitors (five or more meals per week) of fast-food restaurants than low scorers.

But more recent research using magnetic resonance imaging (MRI) scans and other technology shows that the brains of these people actually are different. Thanks to these new technologies, scientists are now able to watch how the brain reacts to food, to photos of food, or just the anticipation of receiving food. If an area of the brain known to house endorphin or dopamine receptors lights up on the screen, scientists are pretty confident the area is awash in brain chemicals.

An increase in these brain chemicals isn't the only thing that can cause overeating, however. Researchers have also discovered that a dopamine malfunction may also play a role. Dopamine is involved in many brain functions, such as learning, memory, and movement. But its role in pleasure may be key to why some folks are so much more susceptible to addiction of any type. "Some people may not produce enough dopamine or their dopamine receptors aren't fully functional, so it takes a lot more ice cream, French fries, or other foods to give you that buzz or satisfaction," explains Dr. Fulton. In a sense, their wiring is "undercharged." The same thing happens to people who abuse drugs or alcohol.

This faulty dopamine response may be inherited, or it could be the result of overeating. The overeating theory goes like this: When you first started overeating, the brain originally reacted by firing lots of dopamine. But it can do that for only so long. Then either the levels decline or the brain doesn't react to them as intensely. So you wind up with less of a rush than before.

It's possible that you could have *supercharged* wiring when it comes to opioids and other pleasure-inducing brain chemicals but also be *undercharged* when it comes to dopamine. That probably makes you the most vulnerable to overeating: You're still getting a big rush from food in some areas of the brain, but a normal amount of food isn't satisfying you because of the dopamine malfunction.

One study provides strong proof that you can be both supercharged and undercharged. The experiment compared MRI scans of two groups of girls both before they were given a milkshake and then as they were sipping the drinks. Half the girls were overweight, the other half normal weight. Certain brain areas lit up more strongly among the overweight girls when they were told that a chocolate shake was coming and while they were drinking it. However, the area of the brain responsible for reward and pleasure—and the section that responds to dopamine—exhibited a more tepid response in the overweight subjects than in their lean counterparts.

How can you tell if your wiring is driving you to overeat? Signs include: (1) Thoughts of food dominate much of your day. (2) You find it not only incredibly difficult to resist fattening foods but also get excited just *thinking* about them. (3) You seem to have a much harder time resisting foods than other people do. (4) You're easily swayed by just the smell of food or by seeing food commercials. (5) You feel addicted to food.

If you think you have this abnormal wiring, we'll give you useful strategies for dealing with it in the Nine Step Program, which starts on page 98. And to keep up with this emerging and fascinating research, be sure to check out www.thebestlife.com, where we'll be posting updates on the topic.

YOU LIVE IN A TOXIC FOOD ENVIRONMENT

Even if a cavewoman had the most amped-up brain wiring, odds are she still wouldn't have been a pound overweight. And that's not just because she was burning up calories hunting, gathering, and child rearing; what also saved her figure was that she never had to contend with the likes of a 42-ounce soda, a large order of fries, or a brownie sundae. But today we're under a constant food assault: At the office, you're fending off cookies and minimuffins. Go buy a book, and you're tempted by candy at the checkout. Shopping for furniture? At my local Crate & Barrel, the constant whir of blenders is a reminder that high-calorie frozen coffee concoctions are just a few steps away at the coffee chain lodged in the store.

Just the sheer number of products available is overwhelming, and, remember, variety stimulates appetite. Even in the recession year of 2009, nearly sixteen thousand new food products—mostly cookies, candy, frozen foods, and other processed foods—were introduced. And they sell at bargain prices. Between 1952 and 2003, the cost of food relative to other purchases fell by 12 percent, according to the U.S. Department of Labor.

So you have high-fat foods sold at low prices virtually everywhere you turn. Sounds like a recipe for disaster, but it gets even worse: Portions of these fatty, cheap, and widely available foods are enormous. Compared to 1980, fast-food drinks, burgers, and fries are twice as hefty; muffins, steaks, and burgers are double or triple in size; and cookies are about seven times larger. You'll find megasized containers of cereal, juice, cookies, and other grocery items at warehouse-type stores. (Notice that you rarely see supersized veggies or pumped-up portions of fruit or whole grains at restaurants or in stores.) Even the portion sizes in classic cookbooks like the *Joy of Cooking* have increased. These larger portions (as well as their higher-calorie ingredients) have caused a spike in calories: There was a 63 percent increase in calorie content per serving between the year the book was published, 1936, and the 2006 version. The largest jump happened between 1997 and 2006.

Our bodies are paying a high price for this cheap, fatty, and oversized food. There's an intricate system of hormones, nerves, and brain chemicals in the body, which not only drives us to eat, but also tells us when to put down the fork; unfortunately, this system has been thrown off in the last few decades. It has been well publicized that the percentage of Americans who are overweight or obese has tripled since 1960. Now the majority of Americans—68 percent—weigh too much. "The factors driving us to eat, especially highly palatable foods like sweets and fried foods, can, and often do, override our satiety signals," says the University of Montreal's Dr. Fulton.

In other words, in the face of 6-ounce muffins, Buffalo wings dipped in blue cheese dressing, three-meat pizza with extra cheese stuffed in the crust, and the like, our caveman drive for high-calorie food trumps the weaker signals telling us we've had enough. Foods this rich and caloric were never part of our caveman ancestors' experience—and weren't even mainstays in our grandparents' generation—but are now a part of what researchers have dubbed the "toxic food environment." This food landscape has not only overwhelmed our brain circuitry, it's actually *changed* it in ways that make food even harder to resist. As I explained, researchers suspect that overeating is one of the causes of a blunted dopamine response, which drives people to need more food to feel satisfied.

And that's just what we're doing: eating more than ever. According to a government study, women today are taking in 308 more calories per day compared to 1971, and men are consuming 162 more calories. That might not seem like a lot, but it ends up adding up to an extra 17 to 30 pounds a year. Plus, when you consider that most people significantly underestimate their calorie intake, it's likely we're taking in even more calories than that.

FIND YOUR MOTIVATION

Now that you understand why resisting food and losing weight has been so difficult—thanks to the internal and external forces pushing you to eat—I hope that you'll cut yourself some slack. Instead of beating yourself up for ordering the muffin instead of the oatmeal, you can start working on changing the impulses that drive you toward the muffin. Because now that you know the enemies, you can start outsmarting them. The first step is to come up with a meaningful and important reason for changing your behavior.

To stay motivated, you must truly believe that your efforts are worth it. With a feeling of true purpose, you'll be more motivated to switch off the game show and spend a half hour in the kitchen making dinner. At the mall, it'll be a lot easier to walk right past the Mrs. Fields cookie stand. The sacrifices won't feel as dire. So, as you did in the previous chapter (and will do in the upcoming chapter), think about reasons that are personally motivating to you. Sometimes the initial reason may seem superficial: You want to fit into your old jeans or lose weight for an upcoming class reunion. If that's what gets you to fill your cart with healthy foods or pushes you to try out the Nine Step Program (page 98), that's fine. But to keep up good nutrition habits for life, eventually you'll need to switch to a reason that resonates more deeply with you.

These are some of the reasons that have kept my clients in it for the long haul: They feel better in their skin when they eat a balanced diet and drop weight. They want to be healthier and more energetic for their family and/or career. And they've developed a taste for wholesome foods and truly enjoy their new way of eating. If the latter reason sounds like something only a nutritionist could come up with, read what the two women profiled in this chapter have to say about savoring new tastes! Some of the reasons listed in the Why List below—such as reducing the risk for heart disease and other conditions—are also listed in chapter 2 (about emotional eating) and chapter 4 (about exercise). It's inspiring to realize that you're doubling or tripling your physical or emotional rewards when you tackle all three fronts: exercise, nutrition, and emotional eating. In the blanks at the end, add any other reasons that are personally important. Return to this list when you're battling a craving for fried foods or sweets and could use a motivation boost.

THE WHY LIST: EIGHT REASONS TO GET CONTROL OF YOUR EATING (PICK AT LEAST ONE)

1. You'll regain control over eating, along with your pride and self-esteem. Being ruled by a bag of chips or losing the battle with yourself over whether to eat a cinnamon bun is profoundly demoralizing.

2. You'll trim down without obsessing over calories. When your meals are rich in fruits and vegetables, with a minimum of high-fat foods, and you switch over to whole grains, calories drop automatically. And then when you conquer any addictive eating problems, you'll lose even more weight. Voilà! All without a single calorie counted.

3. You'll open up a new world of tastes. Taste buds that have been battered by hypersweet, salty, and rich foods have a hard time sensing—much less appreciating—more subtle flavors in fruits, herbs, vegetables, a fresh piece of fish, and other natural foods. When you stop eating the hyped-up foods, your taste buds recover, and suddenly a wide world of foods that are lower in calories and not addictive becomes appealing.

4. You'll cut your heart disease risk. In fact, if you pair a good diet with regular exercise, you can slash your risk by up to 80 percent.

5. You'll reduce the risk for type 2 diabetes and prediabetes. A good diet that promotes weight loss can even reverse prediabetes and, in some cases, type 2 diabetes.

6. You'll decrease your cancer risk, sometimes dramatically. People tend to think that cancer is strictly in the genes, but about a third of cancer cases are caused by poor diet (not enough fruits and vegetables, too much saturated fat, red meat, and alcohol), being sedentary, and/or being overweight. (Another third is attributable to smoking.)

7. You'll boost your brain, bone, and eye health. Replacing unhealthy saturated fat with healthier unsaturated fats (see pages 94–95 for examples of each type of fat) may reduce the risk of Alzheimer's disease and other forms of dementia. Loading up on greens, such as spinach and kale, can help protect against cataracts and macular degeneration, a leading cause of blindness. And a diet rich in all types of vegetables and fruits (as well as calcium and vitamin D) is linked with better, stronger bones.

8. You'll protect your children. Jennifer Levanduski, profiled on page 123, explains it perfectly: "It's so important to me to lead by example so that my children learn proper, healthy eating habits to last a lifetime." Many of the mothers interviewed for this book expressed the same sentiment.

Add your own reasons here:

9. _____

_____

10. _____

_____

KILLER CRAVINGS

A big bag of potato chips, a bacon cheeseburger with fries, an oversized chocolate chip muffin; it seems like these foods possess a special power over us. What makes them so irresistible is not one specific ingredient—the salt or fat or sugar—but a killer combination of two or more of these. In fact, food companies have figured out the percentages of fat, salt, and sugar that make it devilishly difficult to stick to reasonable portions, explains Dr. David Kessler, former commissioner of the U.S. Food and Drug Administration (FDA), in his book *The End of Overeating: Taking Control of the Insatiable American Appetite.*

To make matters even worse, food manufacturers have incorporated so many different flavors into their products, which appeal to our drive for variety. Just look at all the Hot Pockets and Hamburger Helper options. (The term *tastes* covers the five basics we talked about earlier: sweet, salty, sour, bitter, and savory. That's just a starting point, though. Flavors, which we experience through the millions of smell receptors in the nose, make it even tougher to stop eating. For instance, that oversized chocolate muffin is made with sugar and fat from the butter, but the addition of the chocolatey flavor from the chips, and vanilla and any other ingredients, makes it even more tempting than a pile of butter mixed with sugar.)

You may know that these foods aren't good for you, but you probably have no idea just how bad they are. For instance, a Burger King Whopper with cheese is obviously fatty—it has nearly a day's worth of unhealthy saturated fat—but did you bargain on getting 63 percent of your daily sodium limit, too? Check out the health risks for each ingredient found in highly craved foods and learn how to limit yourself.

Fat

The risks: In excess, *any* type of fat sets you up for weight gain because fat has more than double the calories per ounce as protein and carbohydrate. But beware, in particular, of two types of fat: saturated fat and trans fat. Saturated fat is found in fatty cuts of beef, lamb, and other red meat; fatty cuts of pork; full-fat dairy products; poultry skin; coconut and palm oils; and sweets made from some of these foods. The main source of trans fats in our diets is man-made: partially hydrogenated oil. You'll find this fat lurking in some brands of margarine, baked goods, frozen foods, and breaded chicken and fish. Fatty beef and full-fat dairy products also contain small amounts of naturally occurring trans fat. Trans fat from any source as well as saturated fat can cause you to pack on dangerous visceral belly fat, which is linked with heart disease, cancer, and more; these fats also clog your arteries, another risk factor for heart disease. Trans fats are the worst of the two because they raise LDL ("bad") cholesterol and decrease HDL (high-density lipoprotein, or "good") cholesterol. In addition, they increase inflammation in the body, which is being shown to be a risk factor for a variety of diseases, from cancer and heart disease to Alzheimer's and arthritis.

Your limit: Aim to consume 25 percent to 35 percent of your calories from fats—that's 50 to 70 grams on an 1,800-calorie diet. Try to make most of your fat (90 percent) monounsaturated (found in olive and canola oils, avocados, almonds, peanuts, cashews, and pistachios) and polyunsaturated (found in corn, peanut, safflower, sesame, and soybean oils, and pumpkin, sesame, and sunflower seeds). Both of these fats have been shown to protect the heart. Also make an effort to include in your diet a particular type of polyunsaturated fat: omega-3 fats (found in walnuts, flaxseed, flaxseed oil, and canola oil, and fatty fish, such as bluefish, mackerel, salmon, sardines, and trout).

Keep your intake of saturated fat to less than 10 percent of your total calories (or 18 grams on an 1,800-calorie-per-day diet). Avoid trans fats or, at most, cap your intake at 1 percent of your total daily calories, which is 2 grams if you're consuming 1,800 calories. You can do this by avoiding sources of trans fat; that means looking at labels and checking the ingredient list for partially hydrogenated oils, and steering clear of foods that contain them. (Any product sporting the Best Life seal as well as Bob's own Bestlife brand foods, including the Buttery Spread, Buttery Spray, and Buttery Baking Sticks are free of partially hydrogenated oil.) And if you avoid fatty beef and full-fat dairy products, you'll have virtually eliminated naturally occurring sources of trans fat.

Added Sugar

The risks: Added sugar, which is any type of calorie-containing sweetener added to a food, such as cereals, cookies, candy, bread, salad dressing, barbecue sauce—even the sugar you add to your coffee or the maple syrup on your pancakes—can be a problem for a few reasons. For one, the main sources of sugar in our diets are soft drinks and other sugary beverages; these have been linked with an increased risk for heart disease and diabetes. Too much added sugar is also associated with high blood pressure, inflammation, and high triglycerides, a dangerous fat found in the blood, as well as a decrease in HDL ("good" cholesterol). Plus, the amount we take in each day (84 grams, or 21 teaspoons) translates to 336 nutritionally empty calories. Naturally occurring sugar—the sugar in fruit and milk, and in small quantities in vegetables—is not a problem because these foods provide many other healthful nutrients and tend not to be addictive.

Basically all calorie-containing sweeteners—white sugar, raw sugar, brown sugar, maple syrup, honey, corn syrup, molasses, fruit juice sweetener, dextrose, or maltose and even high-fructose corn syrup—are about the same healthwise. The only exception is plain fructose, which is being used in products like energy drinks and some foods marketed to those with diabetes, because it doesn't raise blood sugar quickly. Some animal studies, and now a few human studies, suggest that fructose causes a spike in artery-clogging cholesterol and triglycerides, promotes weight gain in the dangerous abdominal area, and increases inflammation, a trigger to a host of diseases. (Agave syrup is 80 percent or more fructose, so in my book, it's basically fructose.)

Your limit: No more than 10 percent of your total daily calories. That translates to about 45 grams if you're taking in 1,800 calories per day. It can be hard to suss out added sugar from naturally occurring sugar because they're not listed separately on the food label. To get an idea of how much added sugar a product has, check the ingredients list. If it contains no sources of naturally occurring sugar (in fruit or milk), or they're way down on the ingredients list, long after added sugars, then you know that most of the sugar is added. And I'd recommend steering clear of all forms of fructose (including the popular "crystalline fructose") or agave syrup until the safety has been established. As the science on sugar and other nutrition issues comes in, we'll post updates at www.thebestlife.com.

Salt

The risks: Foods loaded with sodium can increase your blood pressure. Chronic high blood pressure, or hypertension, is a leading cause of heart disease, stroke, and kidney disease. Another problem with sodium: A high-salt diet can make it harder to give up high-calorie foods. By adding salt to chips, pretzels, sweets, and many other foods, manufacturers increase the foods' addictive powers. And as long as you keep eating these foods, your taste buds aren't going to be satisfied with lower sodium levels. (See "Train Down Your Tastes for Fat, Salt, and Sugar," on page 121.)

Your limit: We do need *some* sodium in our diet; our bodies don't make it, and we can't function without it. (Sodium helps regulate muscles, including the heart, for instance.) But we don't need anywhere near the crazy levels we're getting. "The average American adult takes in 3,734 milligrams daily; studies show that we need only a fraction of that," says Paul K. Whelton, MB, MD, MSc, president and chief executive officer of Loyola University Medical Center. Although some organizations recommend 2,300 to 2,400 milligrams daily for healthy individuals, 1,500 milligrams (the level recommended for people with hypertension) might be a safer bet. In fact, the U.S. government will probably be suggesting in its upcoming *Dietary Guidelines for Americans* that *everyone* cap it at 1,500 milligrams daily. (As of press time, the *Dietary Guidelines* were still not finalized, but odds are that the sodium recommendation will stick.) The recommendations dip to 1,300 milligrams for fifty-one- to seventy-year-olds and 1,200 milligrams after age seventy; that's because you usually need fewer calories as you age, and when you eat fewer calories, you typically consume less sodium.

FORGING NEW PATHS TO PLEASURE

Imagine a life where you feel in control of food. You're eating a balanced diet, calories are in check, and you've left room for occasional treats. You lose weight and feel really good about yourself. You know you're protecting yourself from long-term diseases and setting a good example for those around you—basically, you're able to check off all the points made on the Why List.

How does that scenario strike you? If you've been ruled by food, it probably strikes you as wonderful, but perhaps unrealistic. You might think, *I've been there, tried that. I've cleaned up my diet before but always gravitate back to overeating or addictive eating.* And as much of a relief as it may sound to not have to worry about food all the time, when you think hard about giving up addictive foods, it might also be a little frightening. Deep down, you may actually think, *Food's just too big a part of my life. I lean on it. It's so much a part of who I am, I'd be at loose ends without it.*

It's perfectly normal to have some ambivalence about giving up a habit that's been with you for a while, sometimes a long while. As much as you may hate it, there's a comfort to it: Food is soothing. And it's the known; without it, will you feel uncomfort-

SAVORING THE TASTE OF SUCCESS

Sheryl Savard, a thirty-eight-year-old lawyer and mother of three, had battled with her weight since she was a teen. "I tried Weight Watchers when I was in high school," recalls Sheryl. "But that lasted all of three weeks, at which point I found and inhaled half a chocolate cake." Her first failed attempt at weight loss, combined with a lifetime of watching her mother yo-yo diet, was enough to convince Sheryl that being on a diet meant deprivation, misery, and disappointment. "I had no answers for finding and keeping a healthy body, so I did nothing, and the pounds piled on." By age thirty-four, petite five-foot-two Sheryl weighed in at 181 pounds. Stressed, overweight, uncomfortable, and trying to raise three children while attending law school, Sheryl decided it was finally time to take back control of her life—and her eating.

She joined Bob's website (www.thebestlife.com) and started revising some long-held beliefs about food, dieting, and weight loss. "It was interesting to realize that even though I claimed to love food, I rarely slowed down enough to appreciate it," Sheryl reflects. "I've adopted the fine art of slow eating, and this has helped me truly enjoy food. And once I learned to savor every bite, some of my favorite foods fell off my list completely. For example, I haven't eaten fast food in almost three years and can honestly say that I don't miss it."

able? If you change your eating habits and then return to your old ways, will you feel even more defeated than you do now? As you did in the previous chapter, you can get a barometer on your readiness to change as well as why you may be resistant to change by interviewing yourself, using the motivational interview in appendix 5. I'm hoping this interview will reveal at least a little willingness to try the Nine Step Program, below.

THE NINE STEP PROGRAM

If you want to stick with a nutritious, calorie-appropriate diet, you're going to have to override some of your brain circuitry and get rid of those automatic impulses to eat when you're triggered by situations or emotions. For instance, maybe you develop a

Now she makes an effort to cook at home regularly, and this has opened a door to new tastes. "I've learned that buying good quality foods and produce, and reading labels, is well worth the cost and effort; 'processed' is just not an option anymore," she says. And while treats are still part of her diet, Sheryl has learned to make smarter decisions with these, too. "I still enjoy my favorite foods but in smaller portions and less often," she explains. "For example, I love chocolate-peanut-butter ice cream, but instead of a double-scoop waffle cone every week, I now eat a child-sized cup on occasion. I have a small piece of dark chocolate or a cup of hot cocoa made with water instead of an entire milk chocolate candy bar. Fruit is now my family's preferred dessert, and for my birthday, we had angel food cake with fresh strawberries."

The changes show; Sheryl is not only forty-six pounds slimmer, but she also became hooked on exercise, recently finishing her first half marathon. Her family is also reaping the benefits. "Bob's program has become so much more than just a weight loss strategy," she says. "The psychological component of looking at your life and assessing what's working and what's not has strengthened our family and other relationships. My husband and I set aside a night each week to focus on long-term and short-term goals."

new MO when you enter the mall: Instead of smelling the cinnamon rolls and battling with yourself over whether to have one (and usually giving in), you take a brisk walk to the opposite end and back. Now *mall* starts to be linked with *walking* in your brain.

The goal of this plan is to break the old habits—eating too many high-calorie foods—and create new, benign, or healthful habits. Because the pathway in the brain from trigger to treat is well worn and, literally, the path of least resistance, breaking the habit may prove tough. You'll probably slip up here and there; that's a normal part of the process. Keep at it, and you'll find that you're giving in less and less and feeling more and more in control. And that's such a good feeling, you'll be coming back for more.

A note about exercise: Do it! By boosting mood, it will make this Nine Step Program easier. And don't worry that exercise will make you even hungrier; the calories you're burning more than compensate for the extra calories consumed as a result of any increase in hunger. And besides, I've noticed that when people start exercising more, their cravings diminish and they gravitate more toward healthier food. (Sushi or a salad is more appealing after a workout than a heavy, fatty meal.) Plus, exercise can help you get back in touch with your appetite signals, which is part of the plan.

Many of these nine steps will be easier to tackle with some support. For instance, a phone call to a level-headed friend can avert a binge; an after-dinner walk with a neighbor can help break your evening ice-cream-and-television habit; going out to eat with your spouse or friend who enjoys healthy food will make it easier to choose well at restaurants. In chapter 2, Ann offers great tips for building a support system.

Step 1: Address Emotional Eating

Feeling out of control around certain foods isn't necessarily an emotional eating problem, but it might be. If you're using food to cope with stress and emotions—both good and bad—you're going to have to work on conquering that problem. People who are able to maintain weight loss report very low levels of emotional eating, according to studies, while people who gain back the weight have a high prevalence of emotional eating. The message is clear: *If you don't conquer emotional eating, you'll never lose weight or keep it off.* In the previous chapter, Ann helped you tackle the problem from all sides. It's a good idea to simultaneously use the exercises in that chapter *and* this treatment plan together. They reinforce each other.

Step 2: Keep a Food Record

You need to know the full scope of your challenge: what you're eating and drinking, how much, when, and in reaction to what triggers. This *invaluable* information will help you in many other stages of this treatment program. The only way to get this information is to log it. If you're a veteran food logger, and it helped you, you understand how powerful this tool is. If it didn't, you may be thinking, "Not again!" But I'm going to challenge you to try again; if your food log wasn't helpful in the past, it's probably because you weren't ready to accept what it told you. Your Lifestyle Log is in appendix 1. (You can print out extra copies at www.thebestlife.com/motivation; you don't have to be a member to get access to the log.) Ideally, you'd log every day for the next month. If you can't, then log as many days a week as you can, with a minimum of four, including two of your days off. Don't worry, you don't have to do it for life! This program requires some intense work up front for results, but it does get easier. And remember, even after you regain control over your diet, your log is always there for you when you need a reality check or a motivation booster.

Step 3: Make an Eating Schedule and Stick to It

People who have a good diet and who are in control around food can be more flexible about when and what they eat. Guided by hunger and fullness signals, they can tell, for instance, that they're still a little full from a bigger-than-usual breakfast and will have lunch an hour later than normal. But when you're giving in to cravings and overeating, your hunger and fullness signals get out of whack. To reset them, you'll have to impose an eating schedule and strictly adhere to it. This is a strategy I picked up from Christopher Fairburn, MD, who heads Oxford University's Centre for Research on Eating Disorders. His book *Overcoming Binge Eating* was published in 1995, and a 2010 study from the Kaiser Permanente health care system supports its effectiveness. Even if you're not bingeing—but instead eating throughout the day—this strategy will help you bring back balance.

Here's what to do: Set up times to have breakfast, lunch, dinner, and one or two snacks. If you've lost touch with your hunger and fullness cues, then *eat the meals and snack(s) whether you're hungry or not*—eventually your body will adjust to your new eating schedule and the signals will kick back in so that you'll find yourself hungry at mealtimes. If you are already in touch with your hunger and fullness cues and you're not hungry at mealtimes, then eliminate a snack or two and/or make your meals a little lower in calories. If you find that you're not hungry because you've been giving in to cravings between meals or you doled out too much food at the previous meal, then stick with the schedule and, at meals, try to avoid eating to the point of feeling stuffed. In the Lifestyle Log, there's a column to track your hunger using a 1-to-10 Hunger Scale, explained on page 230. You'll refer to this column to determine how often you eat in response to hunger (if you even feel the sensation). You know you're getting better when you start seeing more 3s and 4s before mealtimes—those numbers correspond with feeling hungry but not starving.

Eat enough; don't diet. Yes, you want to lose weight, but this isn't the time to start significantly cutting calories. At this point, you have a much bigger problem than your excess weight—your food addiction—so it's best to focus on this first. After all, not eating enough only makes you more vulnerable to your addictive foods. So make sure your meals are satisfying and that you're taking in enough calories. Landing the right calorie level involves a little trial and error; you know you're in the right zone when, except for just before mealtimes, you're not *physically* hungry (which, I know, is a sensation some of you need to regain) and you have enough energy to exercise. For most women, that means not going below 1,700 calories; for men, at this exercise level, no lower than 1,900 calories. I realize that these calorie levels may seem high if weight loss has been your focus, but, again, your focus shouldn't be on weight loss right now. So use these numbers as a starting point and work up from there if necessary. (To see what balanced days look like at these and other calorie levels, check out the meal plans in any of the three *Best Life* books or visit www.thebestlife.com, where you'll also find hundreds of recipes, each complete with its own nutritional analysis, and discount coupons for Best Life products.)

Still, you don't want to overeat; that just reinforces the bad eating habits we're trying to break. So be sure to get the most filling and appetite-quelling meals for the calories. Check out the "Keep It Satisfying" box on the next page.

Write down your schedule on the following page. Eat as close to the assigned times as possible—ideally, within thirty minutes. Have at least one healthy snack, such as a tablespoon of peanut butter or a slice of reduced-fat cheese on a few whole grain crackers, or a piece of fruit and a few tablespoons of nuts, or a slice of turkey on a small piece of whole grain bread spread with reduced-fat mayonnaise. If two or three snacks prove an even better deterrent to caving in to the addictive foods than one snack, then have more snacks and eat a little less at mealtimes.

MEAL	TIME OF DAY (MEALS SHOULD BE NO MORE THAN FOUR HOURS APART)
Breakfast	_____
Snack *	_____
Lunch	_____
Snack *	_____
Dinner	_____
Snack *	_____

* Have at least one healthy snack; more if helpful.

KEEP IT SATISFYING

It's easier to quell a craving when you're not hungry. So, along with sticking to an eating schedule (step 3), eating "high-satiety" meals—meaning those that satisfy hunger long after you've left the table—can also help take a bite out of hunger.

High satiety does *not* have to mean high calorie. In fact, many high-satiety foods actually help you lose weight. While your body requires a certain number of calories every day to keep you satisfied and minimize hunger, it's also looking for that satiating sensation of a full (but not overstuffed) stomach. When the stomach stretches to accommodate a meal, nerves relay a "full" signal up to the brain; that usually takes about 20 minutes from when you start eating. That's where the volume (how much space a food takes up) and the weight of a meal or snack come into play. It turns out that you eat about the same weight of food every day (the actual weight differs from person to person). So if you hit that weight with lower-calorie foods, you'll be just as satisfied as if you filled up on high-calorie foods, given, of course, that you're meeting your basic calorie needs. For instance, have a cheese Danish and a cup of whole milk for breakfast, and you've consumed about 11 ounces of food (approximately 2 $\frac{1}{2}$ cups) for 411 calories. But for that exact same number of calories, you could have had 1 cup of cooked oatmeal topped with 2 tablespoons of chopped walnuts and 1 teaspoon of maple syrup, served with 1 cup of strawberries and 1 cup of fat-free milk—for double the weight, 22 total ounces. The second breakfast weighs twice as much as the first, and if you were to measure it in cups, it's about a third larger. Clearly, the latter breakfast will be more satiating for the calories.

Wondering how the weightier breakfast contains the same number of calories as the lighter one? The answer is simple: It contains more water. Water is heavy, and watery foods are bulky and help make a meal satiating. Strawberries are 91 percent water, similar to most other fruits and vegetables. Fat-free milk is 90 percent water, and even the oatmeal is 83 percent water. A cheese Danish, on the other hand, is just 31 percent water, and while the whole milk is 88 percent water, it has nearly double the calories of fat-free milk because of all the fat.

So here are the ingredients you'll need to create satiating—but calorie-controlled—meals and snacks:

- Water-rich foods such as fruits, vegetables, and low-calorie (broth-based or vegetable puree) soups. About half your plate should be fruit and/or vegetables at each meal. And starting off with 100 calories of a low-calorie soup can make it easier to stick to a reasonable calorie count for the entire meal.

- Fiber-filled foods such as (again) fruits and vegetables, whole grains, bran-based cereals, high-fiber crackers (such as Wasa crispbread) and wraps (such as whole wheat tortillas and Flatout Flatbread), and beans (legumes). The fiber component of these foods is calorie free and expands in the gut, creating a sense of fullness. If you struggle to meet your daily fiber goal (at least 25 grams for women and 38 grams for men), and need a boost, you can try a fiber supplement, like Benefiber.

- Protein is particularly satiating, and keeping it lean helps you cut down on calories and artery-clogging saturated fat. You don't need much: just 2 to 4 ounces per meal. Eggs and liquid egg whites (such as Better'n Eggs and All Whites), fish, skinless poultry, pork tenderloin, and tofu are good choices. Because red meat is linked to certain types of cancer, limit even lean cuts of red meat to once a week. Milk and soy milk are rich in protein, so they cover your protein needs for breakfast. And if you're looking for nutritious vegetarian sources of protein, you can go for tofu, lentils, legumes (such as black beans and pinto beans), or one of the many Best Life approved gardein products.

▪ Low-glycemic-index carbohydrates can help suppress hunger. The glycemic index (GI) is a 1-to-100 ranking of the extent to which a set amount of carbohydrates raises blood sugar. Foods with a low glycemic index (55 and under) elicit the slowest and smallest rise in blood sugar, followed by medium GI foods (56–69) and high glycemic index foods (70–100). So, ideally, most of your carbs will fall into the low or medium levels. Most fruits and vegetables are low GI. Milk and yogurt are as well, because protein slows the journey of the digested food to the gut. But it varies when it comes to grains; here are some lower-GI grain choices:

> Barley
> Bulgur wheat (cracked wheat)
> Oatmeal (the thicker the cut, the lower the GI; steel-cut oats are best)
> Pasta (including regular pasta, whole grain pasta, and pasta enriched with fiber
>   and/or protein such as Barilla Plus)
> Wheat berries

In *The Best Life Guide to Managing Diabetes and Pre-Diabetes,* you'll find the glycemic index of many more foods, because a low-glycemic-index diet helps manage these conditions. You can also look up the GI of foods on www.glycemicindex.com, a website maintained by the University of Sydney's Human Nutrition Unit, School of Molecular Bioscience.

▪ Fat boosts satiety by helping slow the passage of food from the stomach to the intestines. Make the healthy fats listed on page 94 your staples. About two fat servings at each meal should do the trick; a serving is about 45 calories, such as 1 teaspoon of oil or 2 teaspoons spread such as Best Life Buttery Spread, or 1 tablespoon of light mayonnaise or nuts.

Step 4: Change Your Inner Dialogue

To overcome food's strong pull and to start rewiring your brain, you're going to have to change some long-held views and ways that you talk and reason with yourself. Instead of telling yourself that you're weak, out of control, and need food, here are new approaches.

- Rethink deprivation. You're going to be cutting back on fattening fare, which has become a big part of your life. Your challenge is to do this without feeling so deprived that you focus even *more* on the foods and go rushing back to them. Just as turning to these foods became a habit you learned, turning away from them is also a learned habit. "Like any good habit, the more you do it, and the more rewards it brings, the more ingrained and natural it will become," says Adrian Brown, MD, a psychiatrist specializing in eating disorders and an associate clinical professor at Georgetown University Medical Center in Washington, DC. "At first, people don't see how cutting back on foods can be rewarding, but if they're persistent, they soon understand. The sense of pride, control, and accomplishment—and usually weight loss—become worth the temporary discomfort of not devouring a doughnut. However, it takes a while to make that switch."

- Agree to handle a little discomfort. While the rewards of passing up high-calorie foods eventually trump whatever difficulties you may experience, how do you deal with the initial discomfort, which can be very agitating? "It's a fine line," says Dr. Brown. "You don't want to set food rules so rigid that you panic or rebel, but you also don't want to completely let yourself off the hook so you're able to continue your behavior. Make an agreement with yourself that you'll accept some discomfort. Go for the easiest sacrifices first, such as not trying out the new ice cream–topped French toast concoction advertised at the pancake house. Or ordering a small serving of fries rather than a larger one. Adjust to these changes first, then tackle the harder, more ingrained habits, like that latte and cookie you have every day at eleven in the morning," suggests Dr. Brown.

- Give addictive foods a mental makeover. Contemplate one of the foods that holds such sway for you. Let's say it's a German chocolate cupcake. What are your immediate associations? Yummy, comforting, exciting, scary, powerful, fattening, loss of control—both good and bad associations might come to mind. Your goal is to break, or severely weaken those associations, so that the cupcake becomes a much more neutral object that no longer has a grip on you. Try looking at it through the eyes of a space alien: It's a dark brown and light brown mound composed of mainly sugar, flour, and butter. It can raise blood sugar and cholesterol, induce guilt and disappointment, and, if eaten when you're not hungry, can make you uncomfortably full. By looking at your problem foods with fresh eyes, they might not look so great anymore. For me, it's Buffalo chicken wings; I view them as little hunks of skin and fat dipped in even more fat!

- Imagine the problem food is not always available. Usually your craving reaches fever pitch only when you know the food's available. You're walking on a boardwalk and start craving fries because there's a French fry stand every few yards. Every afternoon the bell in your head goes off at three o'clock for a candy bar from the vending machine just one floor down from your office. When you're lying in bed, you might be thinking about the cookies in the cupboard, but you're probably not having an overwhelming craving for the bacon-stuffed potato skins at the T.G.I. Friday's fifteen miles away. So your mental trick is to tell yourself that foods that are physically within your reach are simply not available, or at least not all the time. It's like going to a museum: The objects are there, but you can't pick them up and take them home. The museum idea has not only helped me say no to unhealthy foods but has also saved me a heap of money I might have spent on clothing or furniture I didn't need.

- Remind yourself that you'll never regret it. "We've all regretted ordering that triple-chocolate mousse cake dessert when we're already stuffed, but rarely

does anyone who skipped it say the next day, 'Geez, I wish I'd ordered it,'"
Dr. Brown points out. "Quite the opposite: You feel elated that you dodged
the calorie bullet. As you're experiencing the craving, give yourself a few
moments to imagine the regret you're going to feel if you eat it and how good
you'll feel if you pass it up."

- When you do indulge, eat mindfully and enjoy. You may have heard the term
mindful eating, which is basically the act of focusing on your food when you eat.
You'll get a lot more satisfaction from eating 100 calories of a food you really
enjoy (in my case, dark chocolate) if you savor it without distractions than if
you scarfed down 500 calories of chocolate or other treats while you were trying
to break up a fight between your kids or racing to get to a meeting on time.
Some people purposefully distract themselves while they're eating problem
foods because they feel guilty about it, so they try not to focus on what they're
doing. According to therapist Angela Taylor, "A lot of my clients have benefited
tremendously from mindful awareness exercises. For instance, I recommend a
'first-bite meditation': Before taking the first bite of food, take a deep breath in
and out. Then take a good look at the food before eating it, smell it, and as it
hits your tongue, concentrate on its tastes, flavors, and textures."

- Drop black-and-white thinking. You know the mentality: You're either being
"good," "on a diet," and ultracontrolled—often depriving yourself of any
foods you like—or you're being "bad," "off the diet," and splurging like crazy.
It's what psychologists call "dichotomous thinking," and it usually stems from
a perfectionist mentality: "If I can't be 'perfect'—for instance, eat only highly
nutritious foods and never exceed my calorie limits—then I'll just give up and
lose total control over my diet." For some people, just a few pieces of candy
are enough to throw them off.

    To help change this mind-set, start by changing the diet rules: A
"perfect" diet isn't one that's devoid of chips and candy and such but one

that allows for indulgences in moderation. That'll keep a few pieces of candy from derailing you. But what if you overdo it big-time? Instead of throwing in the towel, tell yourself, "Yes, I overate. Overeating happens, it's a normal part of life. It happens to thin people and to people who successfully keep their weight off. It makes no sense to punish myself for overeating by giving up on a healthful diet and gaining weight. Instead I'm going to respect my body and go right back to healthy eating." The simple act of brushing your teeth can help you transition out of overeating mode and put you back on track. On days that you overeat, you can work off some of those extra calories by getting more exercise, but if you can't, then don't worry about it. Otherwise you might fall into another perfectionist trap: "I didn't burn off the calories, so I might as well quit my fitness program." And try to put your overeating episode in perspective. How many calories was it, really? Remember, it takes about 3,500 *extra* calories—on *top* of your regular calorie needs—to gain a pound of fat. Odds are you didn't overdo it by that much, and even if you did, you can lose a pound. It'll take a little effort, but it's not a catastrophe. Examine your overeating episodes carefully: What was the trigger? How can you plan better next time to avoid it? That's what step 5 is all about.

Step 5: Have a New Plan A

When it comes to dealing with addictive foods, the internal battle usually goes something like this: You get a craving, argue with yourself over whether to give in, and, most likely, give in. You've probably engaged in that debate at the worst possible places: at the coffee shop, staring at the cookies in the display case, or standing at the door of a fast-food joint or other tricky spots. But with a plan in place, you're less likely to have temptation staring you in the face. Now imagine that you've planned in advance to have a cookie at the coffee shop twice a week: on Monday and Friday. Just the act of planning—setting boundaries for yourself—means that it will be a lot easier to stay away from the coffee shop the remaining days of the week. Or your new fast-food plan might be that you don't have fast-food breakfasts, period, but can go three times a week for lunch and choose from three different items all under a certain calorie level. Like these examples, make your plan very specific: which foods you'll eat, how much you'll eat, and when you'll eat them. Your plan might mean that you're still eating too many fattening foods, but that's okay for now. As you gain more control, you can cut out more and more of these foods.

"Planning is a very important way of combating our toxic food environment," explains Dr. Brown. "You decide what's going to happen, you take control, you are not buffeted by the forces of baked goods brought into your office or the special on the menu. You're planning for success." It may not be enough just to carry the plan around in your head. "Taking a strategy from the well-known cognitive therapist Judith Beck, I suggest to my patients that they write their plan down on note cards or type it into their smartphones. They carry around the written plan to pull out when the situation arises. Reading it brings them back to their earlier conviction, to their health goals, and raises the stakes for sticking to the plan," she says.

On a piece of paper, on note cards, or in your phone, start coming up with new strategies to deal with cravings and situations that leave you vulnerable. You can use the format below as a guide. (I recognize that the "old approach" might be your current approach, but let's think positively that it *will* be a thing of the past!)

TYPICAL TRICKY FOOD SITUATION	OLD APPROACH	NEW STRATEGY

In addition to writing it down, here's another way to reinforce your plan. Visualizing the plan in advance has proved helpful to many people: It's like producing a thirty-second movie in your head. Athletes use this same visualization technique before a game when they imagine themselves scoring a goal or hitting the game-winning shot. Or a job candidate might run through a successful interview in her head while she's waiting in the reception area.

For this exercise, choose a time when you have a few free minutes. Sit down, relax, close your eyes, and imagine yourself in a typical tricky food situation. For instance, let's say that you're coming into work and approaching the lobby kiosk where you always stop to buy a bag of chips. Now, in your mind's eye, see yourself successfully enacting your plan: passing the kiosk, not even slowing down, then heading up the staircase to your office. Give your minimovie color and a sound track. What are you wearing? What are the sounds of the lobby? Did the kiosk employee call out to you? How did you respond while still walking by? The more vivid the image, the stronger a tool it will be. Practice conjuring up this vision until it becomes very easy to access. The next time you're in the lobby and those chips are calling out to you, instead of listening to them, pull out your visualization—it will help fortify you to just keep on walking. Now do the same for similar situations.

Along with your specific plans for specific situations, also come up with alternative activities you can do anytime. Cravings don't last forever, so if you can ride them out while doing something else, odds are they'll pass. I know this well. Five times out of ten, when I start walking to the chocolate shop down the street, by the time I arrive, the craving has passed. I'll either turn back and walk home, or I'll buy a bar and have a piece of it later, when I'm ready to fully enjoy it. (I wouldn't have been able to have chocolate lying around before, but one of the joys of following the nine steps is that you gain control over food. And keep in mind, it's perfectly okay to have treats on this Nine Step Program; in fact, it's encouraged to prevent deprivation. See step 6 for details.)

Think of things you can do when a craving strikes and you're not physically hungry or it's not time to eat a scheduled meal or snack. Ann offered some great choices in the previous chapter. I've also mentioned some of them on the following pages; they're such lifesavers that it can't hurt to read them twice! *Don't be discouraged if they don't work as well as food at first.* Remember, the circuits in your brain connecting the scent of a

Cinnabon to eating one, or your afternoon break at the vending machine and other food connections, are well worn and comfortable. Replacing them, even with activities you enjoy, may not be as satisfying at first. Keep at it, and you'll eventually carve out a new, effective groove, one that doesn't involve food.

Ideally, your replacement activity will spark your brain's pleasure centers in a similar manner as food. Those will be the most powerful and quickest for you to adopt. These are activities that soothe and comfort, or give you a little thrill, stimulation, or sensual pleasure. But they don't all have to be that way. There's plenty of evidence that simply distracting yourself even in the most mundane ways can enable you to ride out a craving. Just getting up and pouring yourself a glass of ice water or folding laundry is sometimes all it takes to shake a craving.

Alternatives in the evening. Nighttime is an especially vulnerable period for so many people. You're catching some downtime, possibly the first time all day, and this is where a lot of addictive eating can occur. To make it less of a threat to your healthy-eating plan, make sure to have a nutritious, balanced dinner, preferably with your family or a friend. The sense of bonding and belonging can keep you feeling fulfilled long after the dinner is over. After dinner, there are plenty of other ways to de-stress and find pleasure, such as:

- Getting absorbed in reading, television, or movies. As long as your total TV time is limited (successful weight maintainers watch less than ten hours of TV weekly), there's nothing wrong with taking an hour or two out of your day to watch a movie or favorite show. An engrossing book or magazine, even the newspaper or Web, can keep you away from food. If you've developed strong associations with eating during that time (curling up on the couch with some candy as you watch TV), you'll have to develop an alternative plan, as described earlier.

- Taking a walk in your neighborhood. (Team up with a buddy if it's safer.)

- Having sex. Close down the kitchen, tell yourself you're not going back in until morning, and turn to your partner. You'll hit pleasure centers that even a hot fudge sundae can't touch!

- Pampering yourself. Take a relaxing bath, give yourself a manicure or pedicure, or ask your partner for a massage.

- Cleaning and organizing. It may not be exciting, but as long as it's not stressful, it can do the trick while you're waiting for a craving to pass.

  Now come up with your own activities:

- _____
  _____
- _____
  _____

Alternatives during transition times. You come home from work, or shopping, or the bank, and without consciously realizing it, head straight to the kitchen. At the office, your first stop is the coffee machine. You have a little downtime between connecting flights and find yourself at the airport newsstand buying a candy bar. When transitioning from one place to the next, from one state of mind to another, from one task to a different task, food is often the in-between step. It serves as a reward ("I deserve a candy bar after that long flight"), as a way to get comfortable ("A coffee and a muffin will help me get started on this dreaded report"), and as a way to procrastinate ("I'll just have a scoop of ice cream before dealing with the chores"). Often, you don't even realize you're doing this. A friend of mine, who was an international reporter for *Newsweek* magazine, told me that unless he had a cup of coffee and a cookie, he had complete writer's block and couldn't write the first word of his article.

Try these transitions in lieu of food:

- Come home and turn on some music, take a look at your garden, check the answering machine, or simply sit and relax for a few minutes. Hungry? If not, don't enter the kitchen until you are.

- At the office, use the first ten minutes for the easiest, most enjoyable tasks.

- Whenever possible, take a walk. At the airport, stroll up and down the terminal; at break time during meetings or conferences, walk briskly around the block a few times.

- Meditate or do breathing exercises. Both will help focus you away from food. (For a breathing exercise, see page 65.)

Alternatives while traveling or on vacation. If you're not careful, a trip can become one extended eating tour. To avoid that try the following:

- Bring comfortable shoes on every trip, even a one-day business trip. Plan a walk if possible. On vacations, walking is the best way to get to know new places.

- Plan an active vacation. It's hard to down a bag of chips while you're snorkeling or biking through the countryside.

- Limit alcohol. Remind yourself that vacation, relaxation, and fun are not synonymous with alcohol. There are so many other ways to relax and enjoy yourself: visiting museums, swimming, or going to the movies. You could simply take a moment to reflect on the fact that you're not at the office or doing household chores!

- Plan meals and snacks. While spontaneity is part of the fun of a vacation, you can be spontaneous within a loose structure. Stick with a daily schedule of three meals plus a snack(s), and research restaurants that offer healthful but enjoyable fare. Want to sample the famous local sweets? Plan them into your day by reducing calories at another meal.

Step 6: Cut Out Some Foods and Reduce Portions

Fatty, sugary, and salty foods beget more fatty, sugary, and salty foods. As explained earlier, it's a vicious cycle in which certain foods set off an explosion of feel-good brain chemicals, so you go back for more and get the same reaction. Eventually the chemicals start percolating in your brain at just the *thought* of the food. That thought becomes obsessive, driving you to eat the food, and so on. Use these strategies to wean yourself off these addictive foods:

- Limit variety. In a perfect world, you'd stop eating all your problem foods today. But this cold turkey approach backfires for most people; the deprivation makes these foods loom even larger, dominating their thoughts until they can't take it anymore and give in, having way more than they would have if the food wasn't forbidden.

  I recommend going back to your food record and figuring out which of the unhealthy, highly craved foods you could eliminate with a minimum of anguish. As explained earlier, variety is a trigger for overeating, so allow yourself just one food from each category. If baked sweets are your only unhealthy addictive food category, then pick just one to have this week. There's this little trick we try to play on ourselves: "I'll have just one cupcake, scone, chocolate chip cookie, and brownie—even if I had them all on one day, at least I didn't go through an entire box of cookies." If that sounds familiar, then choose just *one* of those foods to keep in your kitchen or, even better, to go out and purchase as a single item. Bringing in a single serving (in other words, one Fudgsicle from 7-Eleven or a medium-sized cookie from the bakery) is a great control strategy. And even items packaged in single servings, such as the individual Hershey's Extra Dark chocolate squares (which carry the Best Life seal), help tremendously with portion control. If you have more than one category—for instance, baked goods, candy, and chips—then, again, pick one food from each category and stick with that alone this week.

Meanwhile, develop a new plan to deal with each food, using the recommendations under step 5, "Have a New Plan A." Your ultimate goal is to be in control of formerly addictive foods, whether that means eating them on occasion or eating a small portion daily. Most people trying to lose weight can get away with about 150 treat calories a day—I actually recommend this to help prevent feelings of deprivation. There may be some foods that you'll have to completely avoid; they're just too difficult to resist. And as you retrain your tastes away from high-salt, high-sugar, and high-fat foods (step 9), your cravings for them will diminish.

■ Stop stuffing. If you've been stuffing yourself for years and/or eating throughout the day without allowing three to four hours to pass in between meals, you may have lost your sense of hunger and fullness. Don't worry, it's a temporary loss; eating on a schedule (step 3) will help bring back this all-important appetite control mechanism. Another way to coax it back: Eat reasonable portions. Do this and you won't leave a meal overly full. Your stomach will shrink back to normal. (Yes, overeating stretches the stomach, but it will return to its regular size.) And you'll stop associating eating with feeling stuffed. Use the Hunger Scale (page 230) to help pare down your portions.

Step 7: Manage Your Triggers

The goal here is to remove as many triggers as possible. Eating triggers, as I explained earlier, are the things that get you thinking about a specific food—a bakery smell, a mind state (like stress), a location, a time of day, even catching a glimpse of a certain food in your kitchen, to name just a few. And your wiring may be making you particularly sensitive to these triggers. Back to the kiosk example: If there was a way to avoid the kiosk by coming into the building through another entrance, you'd have removed one cue. But if the building itself is one giant cue, then you'd have to use self-talk, planning, and visualizations to help you keep away from the kiosk. You may not even have figured out all your triggers; the "Situation/Emotions" column in the Lifestyle Log might shine a light on some. If stress and emotions are your main triggers, using the worksheets and exercises in "Overcoming Emotional Eating," chapter 2, will be tremendously helpful.

Check out the table below to see if you spot any of your triggers, and try out the advice for unhooking the trigger from eating.

YOUR TRIGGER	HOW TO UNPLUG THE TRIGGER FROM THE FOOD
Problem food or food advertisement	A bag of chips on the kitchen counter is basically an invitation to eat them—same with other problem foods. Spare yourself the temptation by ridding your fridge, pantry, and cabinets of unhealthy trigger foods. It may be okay to keep one treat around if it's part of your plan (see steps 5 and 6). And don't discount the power of food ads; flip the channel or turn the magazine page and get them out of sight!
Time of day (for example, you always have a candy bar at eleven in the morning)	Have *no* food at your trigger hour—or drink water instead. Other than your scheduled meals and snacks, don't tie addictive foods to any particular hour of the day.
Place (kitchen, bakery, ice-cream shop, in front of the TV)	Unless it's written into your plan, avoid the place if possible. For instance, if it's a doughnut shop on your way to work, take a different route. If you must be in the place, then get out as soon as possible. If the kitchen is a trigger, for example, trade kitchen duties for other chores with your family members. If sitting in front of the tube is your trigger, drink water (or another calorie-free beverage), or even better, watch TV while you're on a treadmill or other exercise machine.

YOUR TRIGGER	HOW TO UNPLUG THE TRIGGER FROM THE FOOD
Situation	Vacations, a day at the beach, shopping in the mall, and other situations are often linked to indulgent foods. Create new food rituals in these places: Eat a real (healthy) lunch at the mall instead of stopping at the cookie vendor. And remind yourself of the true reason for your outing: to buy a gift, or to mail a letter, or to get to work.
Stress from being overscheduled	Drop unnecessary activities from your schedule and bolster your support system so that your friends, spouse, or hired help can take on what you can't handle. Meanwhile, start shifting over to nonfood ways of dealing with stress. The previous chapter offers a lot of recommendations on this topic.
Emotions	Using food to cope with emotional pain or turmoil or to celebrate happy times is a particularly hard habit to break, especially if you're the type of person who's wiring makes food particularly rewarding. That wiring, as described earlier in this chapter, means that food gives you a bigger high and/or you have a blunted dopamine response, so you need more food to reach that high. Going through the nine steps in conjunction with the emotional eating exercises in the previous chapter will help you unlink emotions from eating.

Step 8: Eliminate (or Limit) Sugary Beverages

If the word *eliminate* only makes you want them more, then make a pact with yourself to systematically cut back until you have only the occasional soda or other sugary drink as part of a planned treat. If these drinks have become addictive, and even the occasional splurge triggers cravings for more, you may have to stay away from them altogether. Even if you don't feel addicted to them, there's still a very good reason to drastically limit sodas, sweetened iced tea, and other high-calorie beverages: They insidiously pack on pounds by loading you up with calories that don't make you feel full. That 12-ounce soda washing down your pizza tacked on 140 calories to your meal—about the same amount as an extra slice of pizza, but the second slice would have filled you up in a way that a beverage just couldn't. Liquid calories don't register well with the body because they don't have the same satiating effect as solid food. Cavemen didn't go around sipping sweetened beverages, and our bodies still haven't figured out how to deal with them. But these drinks *do* register with your fat cells; those excess calories get tucked away as body fat. As a rough guideline, an extra 140 calories above and beyond your daily needs can add fifteen pounds of body fat in a year's time.

And on average we're consuming way more than a single 140-calorie sweetened beverage per day. In fact, sweetened beverages make up about 21 percent of our daily calories—that's double the percentage in 1965. If you're taking in 1,800 calories, that's 378 calories daily from sugary beverages. The average American drinks 222 *more* beverage calories a day now than in the 1960s, nearly all coming from sugary drinks. We're sipping our way to obesity and other chronic illnesses. In the long-running Nurses' Health Study, which has surveyed hundreds of thousands of nurses about their health and habits since 1976, women who increased their intake of sugar-sweetened beverages over a four-year period gained about eighteen pounds compared to a six-pound gain for women who decreased consumption. It's thought that the increased risk for heart disease and type 2 diabetes from drinking sugary beverages is partly explained by the pounds these drinks put on, and also from their rapidly absorbed sugar, which spikes blood sugar and insulin levels. (Insulin is the hormone responsible for keeping blood sugar levels normal—people with type 1 diabetes stop producing insulin and those with type 2 diabetes either have too little insulin or their cells aren't receptive to the hormone, or both. It's theorized that by constantly stimulating insulin release with sugary and high-glycemic-index foods, the pancreas, which produces insulin, starts to wear out and type 2 diabetes ensues.) Soft drinks also crowd out milk consumption, thus lowering calcium intake.

If sodas weren't bad enough, now you also have to deal with the temptation of Frappuccinos and other blended coffee drinks. When researchers surveyed people buying coffee at fifty-two Starbucks and seventy-three Dunkin' Donuts stores in New York City, they discovered that two-thirds of the coffee cups coming out of Starbucks and one-third from Dunkin' Donuts were blended coffee drinks, which contain an average of 239 calories each.

So, if all that doesn't prompt you to start thinking about cutting back on high-calorie beverages, here's a way to make it more real. Go into your kitchen, get out the measuring spoons, and pour out 12 teaspoons (4 tablespoons) of sugar into a small glass. That's the amount in 12 to 14 ounces of most soft drinks, sweetened iced tea, punches, and juice drinks. Now add 4 more teaspoons—that's the amount in a Dunkin' Donuts large Mocha Spice Latte. That's a lot of sugar!

Next, turn to your Lifestyle Log and circle all the sweetened drinks in one color pen, then all the diet drinks in another color. (You can skip 1 percent or fat-free milk, or soy milk that contains about 100 calories per cup, such as Silk plain or Silk vanilla soy milk. And it's okay to have 4 to 6 ounces of juice daily. Those are part of your basic healthy diet.) How many sweetened beverages or diet drinks are you averaging per day? Are there days that you drink a lot more than usual? Decide how much you can cut back without feeling anxious and deprived. Perhaps you can try starting with 50 percent.

Now come up with replacement beverages. While you might have thought that diet soda or other diet drinks would be a good alternative because they don't contain calories, you may have already figured out (because I had you circle them in your log) that this isn't the case. In fact, I'd recommend them only as a last resort. They may be calorie free, but they're still very sweet, which undermines your efforts to train down your taste for sweets (step 9). Plus, diet drinks perpetuate your associations between *sweet* and *beverage,* making it difficult to drink healthful *un*sweetened beverages. But if the only way to break a regular soda habit is to drink diet soda, then lean on the diet drinks for a while and gradually wean yourself off them. Eventually nearly all diet drinks and sugary beverages should be replaced by the following options:

- Water (your mainstay, comprising at least 80 percent of your beverage intake)

- Sparkling water (plain, or if flavored, no sweeteners, including artificial sweeteners)

- Water or sparkling water with a splash (no more than 2 tablespoons) of fruit juice

- Unsweetened iced tea

- Unsweetened iced tea with a splash (about 2 tablespoons) of fruit juice

- Coffee with a splash of 1 percent or fat-free milk, or black

A note about water: If you're used to flavored beverages, you may be out of the habit of drinking water or have decided that you don't like it. As you move away from sugary beverages, your taste for water should return. In the meantime, try to be creative about ways to encourage yourself to drink more water. For instance, keep a beautiful cup that will inspire you to drink more water on your desk. And set goals for yourself throughout the day—try to hit a certain number of glasses by lunchtime or by mid-afternoon. You can even keep track of your intake online at www.thebestlife.com.

Or challenge yourself to drink more water on the Nestlé Pure Life website (www .nestle-purelife.us), which periodically runs contests, such as taking a pledge to substitute water for a sugared drink each day, with prizes and coupons offered to participants.

Step 9: Train Down Your Tastes for Fat, Salt, and Sugar

Addictive foods tend to have pumped-up flavors, tastes, and textures; think of all that's going on in your mouth when you eat a pepperoni and sausage pizza, or a hot fudge sundae topped with nuts and whipped cream, or even an Oreo, which is not only sweet and chocolatey but also crispy and creamy. It's hard for your average blueberry or orange—or even a really spectacular blueberry or orange—to compete. Their flavors, and those of other fruits, vegetables, and other unprocessed foods, are too subtle for a tongue used to extremes of salt, sugar, and spices. Ditto for fried foods. Even a nicely marinated, tender piece of grilled chicken will lose out to the fried version if fried is what you have a hankering for. "People like what they're familiar with," observes Marcia Pelchat, PhD, a food psychologist with Monell Chemical Senses Center, a scientific institute in Philadelphia dedicated to researching taste and smell. "If you eat cheeseburgers and fries, that's what you'll crave. But if you start eating salad and grilled fish, after a while you'll want that type of food."

And that should come as a big relief; when you let go of your addictive foods, you won't be left high and dry. You'll actually *prefer* the healthier fare in time. But first you have to make that transition to healthier fare. Here's how:

- Scale back gradually. "You could go cold turkey—switch to low-sodium, low-sugar, or low-fat foods tomorrow—and in about a month you'll actually prefer these foods. But I recommend doing it gradually," advises Dr. Pelchat. "It'll take a little longer, but you'll enjoy your food more and be less likely to rebel or give up." So don't go from a tomato soup with 800 milligrams of sodium per cup to one with 60 milligrams; you'll hate it. Instead start buying soup in the 500-milligram-per-cup range and see if you can work down from there. In recipes, cut sodium by about 25 percent, and when you get used to that, keep working your way down until your recipes have no more than ⅛ of a teaspoon of salt per serving. As the rest of your diet becomes lower in sodium, you shouldn't miss the salt in that stew and in other dishes. And if you do, then a very small amount of salt added at the table will do the trick. (See "The Case for the Salt Shaker," on page 125.)

  This gradual approach works well for fatty foods, too. For milk, go from whole to 2 percent and stay there for a week or two. Then mix 2 percent with 1 percent for another week or two. Then take another week or two to get used to just 1 percent. You can stick with 1 percent or train down to fat-free (skim) by mixing the two for a week or two before adjusting to fat-free milk alone. Switching from fatty to lean meats is a little trickier because lean meat can be tough and dry if not cooked properly. If you're a burger fan, I recommend not

TAMING A SWEET TOOTH

Jennifer Levanduski, a thirty-seven-year-old stay-at-home mom, struggled to keep the pounds at bay for most of her childhood and adult life. But during her second pregnancy in 2007, her weight climbed past a dangerous 265 pounds. "After my son was born, my weight came down into the 240s," explains five-foot-nine Jennifer, "but my gelatinous body repelled me. I kept saying, 'I have to go on a diet,' but I didn't really feel the motivation to make a change, and I wasn't ready to give up my sweets." She jumped from one fad diet to the next looking for a quick fix, but, not surprisingly, nothing worked.

Then, in October 2008, Jennifer got an email about a casting call for the Discovery Health Channel to be a part of a series that Bob Greene was hosting called *What's Making You Fat? A Best Life Special.* She answered the email and got selected! "The casting call was an answer to a dream. It put me on a completely new track, which I continued with after the show by joining the online program (www.thebestlife.com). I now eat real meals, don't let myself go hungry, and allow myself moderately portioned treats. This approach ended the diet-deprivation-binge-diet cycle I was on for so long," she explains. "I don't want to get to the point where I tell myself I *can't* have something. Instead I have a portion-controlled amount of the splurge food and log it in my food diary to make myself accountable. It's amazing that after one bite, I often find it disgusting and throw the rest away! This happened recently when I tried an Oreo Cakester. I'd eyed those at the market for months, imagining the chocolatey, fluffy goodness melting in my mouth. What I tasted instead was lard; it coated my tongue and turned my stomach. Into the trash it went!"

A year and a half after taping the show, she had lost seventy-five pounds. And Jennifer is still losing, thanks to exercise coupled with her new way of eating. "Now, to satisfy my sweet tooth, I chew sugar-free gum," she says. "It provides a sweetness and keeps my mouth busy so I can't eat other foods—bonus! I've also rediscovered meringue cookies. I make small ones at home that are only about ten calories each. There are so many ways to vary the flavors of them, too. My favorites right now are vanilla, peppermint, and mini-chocolate chip.

"The Best Life program has allowed me to find balance," says Jennifer. "My new life is so much more rewarding than my old sweet fixes."

even trying to make an extralean burger—too dry. But extralean ground beef works well in chili, Sloppy Joes (there's a great Sloppy Joe recipe in *The Best Life Diet Cookbook*), and other mixed dishes. And lean cuts such as tenderloin and flank steak can be delicious if marinated properly and cooked quickly.

Finally, do the same for sugar: Gradually cut back in recipes like banana bread, cakes, pies, and cookies. (If making desserts at home gets you into trouble, then don't. Instead get a single-serving treat when you go out. Just make sure to check labels and choose sweets with the lower sugar levels.) And with chocolate, the higher the percentage of cocoa, the less sugar it contains. Milk chocolate generally has less than 40 percent cocoa, and dark chocolate usually has 50 percent or more.

■ Meanwhile, pump up other flavors. As you bring down the salt, sugar, and fat, keep food tasty and interesting by infusing it with other flavors. Sodium is the toughest hurdle because, as Dr. Pelchat explains, "People aren't drawn to salt just for its taste—it also brings out flavors in foods, such as those in olive oil and other fats, and it masks bitter flavors." So if you like olive oil, buy extra-virgin (it's more flavorful) and sample a few brands to get one that is deep and intense. And use a heavier hand with herbs, spices, onion, garlic, lemon, and other citrus juices or grated citrus rinds in your dishes. For instance, spare yourself the 960 milligrams of sodium in a serving of Herb and Butter Rice-A-Roni by adding fresh chopped or dried herbs to a half cup of cooked brown rice and tossing with toasted almonds and a dash of salt and olive oil for a mere 160 milligrams of sodium. And if you find that lowering the sodium makes the bitter flavors in greens, like watercress and arugula, emerge too strongly, just mix them with romaine, oak lettuce, or other milder greens.

Fruit is going to be your ticket to weaning yourself off sugary desserts, but strawberries for dessert is a tough sell if you've been indulging in brownies, cakes, cookies, and pies. If it's excellent-tasting fruit, you'll have a much easier time making the switch. One of the Best Life nutritionists sends me Harry and David pears every year, and I get nearly as excited by that package as if she'd sent me a box of chocolates! Here's where farmer's markets really come through for you: The ripe-picked apples, pears, peaches, melons, and other fruits leave most supermarket fruit in the dust. And if you don't have access to exceptional fruit, mixing together a little honey and orange juice and tossing it with chopped fruit does wonders for taste.

THE CASE FOR THE SALT SHAKER

If you're wondering where all the excess sodium in the American diet comes from, don't look at the salt shaker. It's responsible for only about 6 percent of our sodium intake. Instead read the labels of the processed foods you're eating, or check out the online nutrition charts for chain restaurants. That's where the staggering numbers show up.

So I'm going to suggest that you go ahead and use the salt shaker at the table and drastically cut back on processed foods and carryout, and taper the salt in recipes to the levels recommended on pages 96–97. Those few crystals that you sprinkle on your food before taking a bite give you a much stronger salt taste than if you'd added many times more salt into the food while you're cooking. And that salt-sprinkled dish will probably give you even more sodium satisfaction than a high-sodium canned soup or other processed food. In a Monell Chemical Senses Center study, using the salt shaker when eating a low-sodium (1,600 milligrams per day) diet raised sodium levels only 20 percent to about 1,920 milligrams daily—still fairly low.

There's just one catch to skipping salt while cooking and adding it at the table instead. "You'll keep sodium low this way, but it doesn't help you reduce your taste for salt," says Dr. Pelchat. That's okay, as long as you're still able to break your addiction to salty foods. Having some salt on your sautéed zucchini doesn't necessarily translate to craving salty fast food. However, if you're not making any headway, you might try putting away the salt shaker for a while and training your taste for salt way down. Eventually the addictive food might taste unpleasantly salty.

■ Check labels. You may be surprised to find out that there are 250 milligrams of sodium in the cereal going into your bowl (11 percent of your daily max) or 8 grams (2 teaspoons) of sugar in the raspberry vinaigrette dressing in your fridge. While the name Chubby Hubby should be a tip-off, you might not have imagined that just a half cup of this ice cream delivers about 60 percent of your daily saturated fat allotment. Once you start comparing labels, you'll find great-tasting foods with half the sodium, salt, and fat. Expect a little trial and error—not every food will be to your liking.

■ Eat more of the healthy foods you already like. You probably have a number of healthy foods in your repertoire, like shredded wheat (a low-sodium cereal), bananas, watermelon, salad with homemade olive oil and balsamic dressing, and low-fat sweets such as Fudgsicles and fruit bars. Lean on these foods as you work on incorporating even more healthy foods.

ACHIEVE YOUR GOALS

Changing something as deeply rooted as your eating habits requires dedication, determination, and planning. For the planning part of the equation, try this goal-setting worksheet, the same one you used in the previous chapter. Pick a goal, fill out the worksheet, and come back to it in twenty-four hours to make sure you don't need to tweak anything. If it seems to be working out, do it for two weeks; that's not so long that it feels oppressive, but it's long enough to start instilling a good habit. If it's *not* working out, then choose a new two-week goal. Blank worksheets are in appendix 4, or you can download them for free at www.thebestlife.com/motivation.

WHAT YOUR GOAL-SETTING WORKSHEET MIGHT LOOK LIKE

1. **What is my healthy-eating goal?** Find a goal you know you can achieve; nothing overly ambitious. For instance: "Keep a food record for at least four days this week and at least two days next week."

2. **What is the most positive outcome of achieving this goal?** This is crucial: You must be able to name and imagine a benefit. Otherwise this technique won't work. The positive outcome is what drives motivation and infuses meaning. For instance: "The food record will help me assess my diet habits, a critical first step needed before making healthful changes."

3. **What is the main obstacle standing in my way?** For instance: "I don't trust myself to write down everything I eat because I never leave myself enough time, and I'm bad at estimating portions."

4. **How can I overcome the obstacle?** Be very specific, noting the "when" and "where" the obstacle occurs. For instance: "I'll make sure to leave time after each meal to write down what I ate. And when I don't have time, I'll take before-and-after photos with my cell phone or camera, then record it later. That will also take care of the accuracy issue."

5. **How do I prevent the obstacle from occurring in the first place?** Again, be specific about the "when" and "where." For example: "To deal with the lack of time, I'll plan an extra one to five minutes after each meal or snack to write down what I ate or to take before and after shots of meals and snacks."

6. **How, specifically, should I achieve my healthy-eating goal?** This means focusing on specifically when and where it would happen. For example, "This Thursday through Sunday will be relatively calm days, so I'll do it then. I'll carry blank Lifestyle Log pages around with me at all times. I'll also always have my phone and/or a camera with me to snap before and after photos of the meals and snacks. That way, I'll have a photo, so I won't forget, or I can share it with someone who can help me determine portion size."

■ Prepare more meals yourself. If you're not a confident cook or simply got out of the habit of preparing meals, take on the challenge and try out some easy recipes with few ingredients. The *Best Life Diet Cookbook* and www.thebestlife .com are filled with such recipes.

■ Give your favorite foods a healthy makeover. This is important on two levels: It staves off feelings of deprivation and trains your tastes to prefer foods lower in sodium, sugar, and fat so that you might not want to return to the old versions. If you can't find a pre-prepared healthier food out there, try making a leaner, lower-sodium, and/or lower-sugar version yourself.

THE PACE OF YOUR STEPS

Nine steps may not sound like many, but taking even one step toward changing your eating habits can be challenging, especially if you're a food addict. If these nine steps seem too hard to do all at once, then don't. Choose one step and use the goal-setting worksheet for a realistic, doable plan to achieve your goal. Work on one at a time, if that's the most you can handle. Or, if you can swing it, work on two at a time. The goal I've picked as a sample—logging your food intake for a few days—is only a suggestion; you don't have to follow it. But it *is* a good starting point for just about everyone. If you're an emotional eater, I'd start by going to chapter 2 and working on that first (if you've skipped around in this book). As your emotional dependence on food wanes, the other steps in this program will be easier to implement.

As the successful maintainers whose stories dot this book illustrate, it is possible to overhaul your diet. In fact, people do it all the time—people with entrenched food addictions, people who might not be addicted but are abusing food, and people who overeat because that's what they were taught. Sure, we get stuck in a groove, but we all have the power to get out of it. Just keep your reasons for change (pages 91–93) in the forefront of your mind, take this at a realistic pace, and you'll be a better eater next week, and an even better one next month and in the years that follow.

4

CONQUERING
EXERCISE AVERSION

By Bob Greene

WE WERE MEANT TO move. And when we don't, we increase our risk of virtually every known ailment. I'm sure you've heard about a lot of the illnesses associated with sedentary living, among them diabetes, coronary heart disease, hypertension, osteoporosis, and stroke. Beyond that, though, researchers are continually finding new ways that physical activity protects our health. We now know, for instance, that exercise strengthens the immune system in ways that can help the body fight everything from small infections to cancer. In another way, by keeping the body leaner, exercise also helps guard against cancers that are associated with body fat, including cancers of the esophagus, pancreas, colon, kidney, and breast. Lowering body fat is one way that physical activity protects against heart disease and diabetes, too.

All this should be enough to get people in their right minds to the gym, but, of course, lots of perfectly sane people don't even own a pair of workout shoes. The number one reason is that many people simply hate exercise. It is *the* biggest barrier to regular physical activity and, by extension, one of the biggest barriers to long-term weight loss success. If you too hate exercise, it's easy to ignore all the reasons why activity is so vital to your health, and I'll even go as far as to say your happiness. But let me state it simply: You really need to do it. One thing we know for sure is that people who have long-term success are physically active. So even if you don't care about all the health benefits of exercise, if you want to lose weight and keep it off, there's virtually no way around it. *You have to exercise.*

The challenge in front of you is to get past your resistance to exercise, zero in on a way to make it part of your life, and stop making excuses about why you can't be physically active. In this chapter, I'm going to give you a few different ways to accomplish those goals. You'll take a step back and think about the reasons you might be reluctant to exercise, find what you can use to motivate yourself, and, by adjusting your mindset, overcome the obstacles that you perceive are getting in the way of activity. You may never learn to love exercise (though who knows? A lot of former exercise haters do), but you will learn to love what exercise does for you. That was the experience of one woman I met on *The Oprah Winfrey Show,* whom I'll tell you about shortly.

I also want to say a word about why I believe you should begin incorporating physical activity into your life even before you attempt to cut calories. This idea doesn't go over big with many people; most want to begin by changing their eating habits. I really have to warm them up to the idea of establishing a fitness routine first.

This is not just me being an exercise kind of guy trying to convert everyone to my way of thinking. There are solid reasons for diving into exercise before you begin fiddling with your food intake. For one thing, most people have greater long-term success when they begin with exercise, and there are several reasons why. Generally, when you eat fewer calories, your body reacts by slowing down your metabolism to preserve body fat, a defense mechanism that helped your ancestors avoid starvation and is still programmed into your DNA today. Exercise, on the other hand, *boosts* your metabolism by increasing production of enzymes that allow you to process more oxygen. That boost counteracts the metabolic slowdown that comes from calorie cutting and allows your body to shed body fat, just as you'd hoped. What's more, the increase in metabolism you get from regular exercise can last the whole day. Exercising might make you a little hungrier, but, on balance, between the calories you burn while working out and the spike to your metabolism, your workouts will nudge you into a calorie deficit. Interestingly, some research shows that while people who exercise do report an increased appetite, they seem to be satisfied with less food at mealtimes. That's going to make calorie cutting less painful when you do begin reining in your food intake.

Consider, too, that exercise preserves muscle, while cutting calories alone can cause muscle loss. Exercise also boosts your mood and gives you more energy, two things that go a long way toward helping you confront the challenge of making changes on the food front.

Another reason that I encourage you to focus on fitness first is because you can see tangible, more immediate results with exercise, and that's motivating. A firmer body, glowing skin, a better night's sleep, an ease that comes from gaining muscle strength— those are all things that come from physical activity and are all things that can inspire you to take self-improvement up a notch. Many exercisers find that their workouts give them the will to refuse that slice of cake or plate of French fries: They don't want to negate the gains they've worked so hard to make.

EXERCISE AND YOUR EARLY YEARS

While exercise aversion is rampant, it's the rare person who didn't begin life as an active person. Have you ever noticed that, before they reach the age where they become mesmerized by PlayStations and computer games, most kids move nonstop? I was such a kid, though we didn't have PlayStations and computer games back then. But even if we did, I think I would have opted to be doing something active. I loved any kind of physical activity—especially outdoor activity. My parents always had to hunt me down when dinnertime rolled around because I was out somewhere riding a bike or kicking a ball, trying to wring out every last minute of daylight before I had to go in for the night. Because I naturally gravitated toward exercise, I easily made the transition into more structured forms of activity like organized sports and phys ed class. In that way, I was lucky. So many people I've talked to had the opposite experience with formal athletic activities, and it's almost always the reason why they grew up to be exercise-hating adults.

When I speak to groups of people, I often ask them, "How many of you had a bad experience in PE class?" Generally, about half of the audience raises their hands—and those are just the ones who admit it. When I think back on my own school days, I can see that, while I might have been having fun, the seeds of exercise aversion were being sown all around me. Whenever my classmates and I were dividing up into teams to play a game like kickball, I was the kid fortunate enough to be picked early on. But then as the selection process went on, I would watch uncomfortably as some of my nonathletic friends stood there fidgeting uneasily, waiting to learn their fate. Their faces would turn red and they'd avert their eyes, looking as though they'd rather be anywhere else on the planet than in that school yard. I knew they were praying, *Just let me be picked second to last, not last,* because being last, of course, was the ultimate humiliation.

And it wasn't only during the cruel process of choosing up sides that my friends suffered. These were the same kids who, to their mortification, could not perform more than a single push-up or lap around the track. It was tough on them. As I was gaining confidence from being able to shoot a ball through a hoop and boot a soccer ball into a net, a lot of my classmates were *losing* confidence because they couldn't sink a shot or kick a ball in bounds.

The funny thing was that while PE was one thing, recess was another. These same kids who recoiled from sports and took such an emotional beating in gym class would run and jump, play tag, and just generally horse around in a very active way during recess. They liked moving; they just didn't like the phys ed teacher telling them what to do or criticizing them for not being fast, agile, or coordinated enough. Do you see what I'm getting at? It's quite possible that even if you weren't one of those kids who got picked early for teams, and even if you think that you've always hated exercise, there was probably a time that you actually loved to move your body.

As we become adults, we have a lot going against us when it comes to physical activity. It gets harder to run or swim or bike or even take a long walk with age, partly because we're not used to it. Life happens, and we can't spend all the time we once did out on the playground running around. (Now kids barely have time to do that either, and forty-eight states don't even require PE anymore, but that's another story.)

Lack of exercise, though, goes beyond lack of time. We don't *have to* move anymore. Elevators. Escalators. Email. Most housing developers don't even bother to put in sidewalks anymore. People who want to walk in these new neighborhoods have to take their chances with traffic in the street. No wonder so many drive everywhere instead. Everything is so automated nowadays that you don't even have to use your hand to open a can or sharpen a pencil anymore. As a result, because so few of us are physically active in the course of everyday living, exercise becomes even more uncomfortable than it might be otherwise. Most people don't find all that panting and sweating pleasurable.

When you add physical discomfort to the bad memories of Coach Woodcock yelling at you for dragging your feet on the track or being late for PE class, you've got layer upon layer of reasons for not getting up off the couch. Still, even with all that going against you, you can relearn to like moving your body or, at the very least, be able to tolerate grinding it out. And I don't know anyone who doesn't like the way they feel *after* finishing a workout.

CHANGING YOUR MIND ABOUT EXERCISE

Not long after *The Best Life Diet* was published, I asked a few people to join the Best Life Diet Challenge on *Oprah*. As they adopted the principles of the plan, the show followed their progress. One of those people was a young woman named Tracy Ring. Tracy was one of the most exercise-averse people I had ever met. The first day, she let it be known that she didn't really see herself exercising; I could barely get her to walk on a treadmill! I was worried. I knew there was little chance that she would succeed if she didn't change her attitude about exercise. But as the challenge went on, Tracy amazed me. She not only did very well, but in a huge turnaround, she became an avid exerciser.

Tracy is someone whose relationship with exercise echoes everything I just talked about. When Tracy joined the challenge, she weighed about 240 pounds. Nine months later, she had lost 74 of them, and now, two years down the road, she has kept the weight off. Exercise played a big role in Tracy's turnaround, something she couldn't have predicted before she made the commitment to lose the weight once and for all.

Tracy, who's now thirty-two, is one of those people I talked about earlier who had a negative experience with activity in her formative years. Grade school, middle school, high school—she found PE awful every step of the way. "I didn't like that you had to change clothes in the locker room and pretend to be cool while feeling self-conscious," she remembers. "Then there is an immediate stratification of who's good at PE and who is not. The good kids rise to the top, and the gym teacher thinks they're fantastic. Sports never came easy to me, but other things like band and debating did, so why in the heck would I kill myself exercising when I was better at other things?" For Tracy, there was also the added pressure of having parents who are extremely athletic. Her dad was on the U.S. Olympic Committee for track and field and is a triathlete; her mother runs marathons.

To hear Tracy talk about her early experience with physical activity, you'd never think that she was the same person who, when I caught up with her recently, had gone to the gym at four-thirty that morning; she had to be at work by seven and didn't want to miss her workout. Despite the fact that she travels about 250 days a year for her job—"My life is like the movie *Up in the Air,*" she says, referring to the film starring George Clooney as a perpetual airline passenger who lives out of his suitcase—Tracy exercises almost every day. She's completed a minitriathlon and regularly enters 5K races. "I wouldn't say I love exercise," says Tracy, "but I do love the way it positively impacts my life."

So how did she go from gymphobic to someone who rises before the sun to get in a workout? When Tracy joined the Best Life Challenge, a friend asked her, "If you're not going to do it now, when millions of people are watching you, then when?" The question struck a chord with her, but it would be wrong to think that she was letting an external factor—Oprah's large TV audience—drive her. (And the fact that Tracy has kept the weight off for two years without an audience to prod her is testament to that.) Tracy's real motivation came from within. "I knew that I wouldn't be happy being a size twenty for the rest of my life," she says. "I had spent years trying to shortcut the system, but I could see that wasn't going to work anymore."

Tracy had found her motivation, which, as I discuss in detail later in this chapter, is an essential part of getting physical activity into your life. But that wasn't all she needed to move forward. There were obstacles in Tracy's life—not to mention her intrinsic dislike of physical activity—that she would need to surmount. The first challenge: making exercise bearable and even somewhat enjoyable.

Tracy has a business degree and is very analytical. She likes facts and figures, and, to her, exercise has become something of a numbers game. She wears a heart rate monitor and tracks how many calories she burns, she sets distance goals (this is where training for an event like a 5K can help), and she checks to see that her energy expenditure through exercise is high enough to balance the amount of food she's eating. It keeps exercise interesting for her. "And it keeps me honest," adds Tracy.

One of the things that most impresses me about Tracy is that she has kept exercising despite her travel schedule. One way she's made that happen is by always staying at a hotel that has a gym, and if she has to miss a workout because of work priorities, she makes it up on the weekends. She even has a good strategy for watching her calories while living out of a hotel room: Before Tracy hits the gym, she orders a healthy meal from room service so that when she gets back, it's there waiting for her, ready to subdue her appetite and keep her from rummaging through the chips and nuts in the minibar.

While getting the logistics down has been no small feat, I think what has most helped Tracy stay committed to exercise is her attitude. It has changed dramatically. Where she may have once resigned herself to any barrier that kept her from exercising, she now finds solutions to the problems. She doesn't make excuses. She doesn't let herself off the hook. If she can't go to the gym, she knows she can always put on a pair of running shoes and jog around her neighborhood. When she's feeling stressed out and lethargic, she reminds herself that she will feel less stressed if she exercises. "It's kind of like when you're sitting at home on the couch on a Saturday night and you don't feel like doing anything, but then you rally, get dressed, put on some makeup, and go out. You're always glad you did," says Tracy. "Exercise is the same way. Afterward, you always feel happy you did it."

When I first met Tracy on *The Oprah Winfrey Show,* she was starting to experience some problems in her marriage. Since then, she and her husband have divorced. In that way, Tracy is like a lot of people struggling with their weight who also have some kind of underlying emotional issue dragging them down. The two are often intimately connected, and when that underlying issue is resolved, or when you get on the road to resolving the matter, changing your eating and exercise habits become easier. Ultimately, what Tracy really had going in her favor is that she made up her mind that she was done simply accepting things that were making her unhappy: a body that wasn't healthy, a marriage that wasn't working. She pinpointed all the things that she needed to do to improve her life, and, highly motivated, she did them to great success.

GETTING PAST THE DISCOMFORT

When I said earlier that our bodies are meant to move, I meant that literally. Our ancestors, after all, were hunters and gatherers; they didn't have the luxury of sitting still. But we are also genetically programmed to rest when we can, and in this modern life, we can rest our bodies pretty much any time we want. As a result, exercise is uncomfortable. Most people aren't used to it. But even as you do get used to it, there's always going to be some discomfort. There needs to be in order for physical activity to have any payoff. All those benefits of exercise—the positive changes to the heart and lungs, the increase in aerobic enzymes, the strengthening of muscle and bone, the production of brain chemicals that improve mood—occur only when the body encounters physical stress and, yes, feels some discomfort.

So I'm not going to sugarcoat it and tell you that you can walk around the block once at a leisurely pace and be done with it (although, if you're doing absolutely nothing, walking around the block once is a good place to start). For real health and weight loss benefits, you need to raise your heart rate to appropriate levels and push some weights around. To some people, that actually feels good, but if it doesn't feel good to you, you have to find a way to improve your tolerance and embrace the challenge.

The good news is that your physical tolerance for exercise will improve with time. Just like your taste buds adapt when you switch to 1 percent milk after a lifetime of the full-fat version, your body adapts to physical activity, which makes it easier to move. But probably what's more important is that you develop a mental tolerance for exercise, and that involves changing your thinking.

It's crucial, for instance, that you see exercise for the accomplishment it is. I'm sure there have been many instances in your life when you gritted your teeth and pounded something out. Maybe you've worked through rocky patches in a relationship or hung in there when a job wasn't going so well. When you reap the rewards of not giving up, it's a great feeling. Look at exercise the same way. I remember Oprah once telling me that when she first began exercising, she'd be on the stair-stepping machine at the gym, huffing and puffing at the lowest possible intensity level, then look to her right and see the woman on the next stair-stepper barely breaking a sweat, *her* intensity level all the way up to the top. It was disheartening. She kept at it, though, and soon she was up to the second level, then to the third and the fourth. It gave her a great feeling of accomplishment, and she wanted to keep that feeling going.

I also remember that when Oprah and I ran the 1994 Marine Corps Marathon in Washington, DC, I looked back at her when we hit mile twenty-five and saw tears of joy streaming down her face. She still gets emotional whenever the subject of the marathon comes up. And with good reason. It was a fantastic achievement. But Oprah is also the first to admit that her weight ebbs and flows depending on how much exercise she's doing, how she handles emotional eating, and how she balances her personal and very busy work life. The good thing is that, after running that marathon, she knows that she's capable of hitting the "zone": that place where exercise is giving you great health and body weight benefits and making you feel confident and capable.

I don't want to give the impression that you have to run a marathon (or even come anywhere close) to feel as though you've accomplished something. In my view, simply getting to the gym regularly or consistently taking brisk walks and lifting a few weights are great achievements. They should make you feel proud, and when you feel proud, it makes exercising all that much easier to bear. I'll go even further and say that it changes you. When you accomplish something that you never thought you could achieve, it makes you look at the world differently. Suddenly, other obstacles in your life look less daunting, too. That's no exaggeration. Seeing your intensity level on the elliptical machine rise—or noticing any sign that you've made progress—is going to lift your spirits and solidify your belief in yourself.

Changing your mind about exercise and getting past the discomfort is all a process. The rest of this chapter is designed to help you navigate your way through that process. Before anything else, though, it's essential that you zero in on *why* you want to exercise. Clarify your motives so you're not just aimlessly out there doing something with no specific purpose. You're going to have a greater chance of staying committed if you see exercise as a means to an end result that you really desire. The next step is to explore your attitudes about physical activity, which will help you better understand what's gotten in your way in the past. Finally, you've got to own up to the excuses you've been making. If your attitudes toward exercise color the whole picture, excuses fill in the details. Excuses are what prevent you from being active on a daily basis, and I think I've heard every one of them—except a good one. It's time to rethink your justifications for not being active. When you look at them closely, I think you'll see that they don't hold up. You really *can* fit exercise into your life.

FIND YOUR MOTIVATION

Earlier I mentioned that exercising can actually motivate you to improve other behaviors—in particular, your eating habits. But before exercise can motivate you, you have to be motivated to exercise, and that, of course, is the crux of the issue. There are many reasons why you *should* be physically active. But if those reasons don't really matter to you—and I mean matter deeply—then you are not going to stick with exercise. It's critical that you find a reason, any reason, that really resonates with *you*. Not with your significant other, not with your best friend, not with the magazine you subscribe to, not even with your doctor. It has to be something that inspires you and only you.

The importance of a significant motivating factor is something I've seen again and again among my clients. But there is also good research—including a series of studies from Portugal—that shows the value of developing an individualized rationale for exercising. One of the studies divided overweight women into two groups. Both received standard advice on diet and exercise, but only one group was encouraged to go deeper and do some emotional work. That group was introduced to many of the same tools you'll be using throughout this book—the motivational interview, understanding individual barriers, and finding the right type of exercise—all with the aim of developing a very personal incentive for staying physically active. After a year, the group that incorporated the psychological and emotional components lost an average of twelve pounds of body fat, compared to just three pounds for the other volunteers.

The women who developed personal motivations averaged 138 more minutes of exercise per week and 2,049 more steps per day (measured by a pedometer) than the other group. Three years later, they were still getting 86 more minutes of physical activity per week than the group that did no emotional work.

What I find particularly interesting about this research is that it showed that inner motivation is something you can acquire. "Our study shows that people can develop a sense of ownership over their behavior, so their desire to exercise stems from within," says Pedro J. Teixeira, PhD, one of the study researchers and a professor in the Department of Exercise and Health at Technical University of Lisbon. "Sustaining an appropriate level of physical activity over the long run most often doesn't come from complying with your doctor's orders or other external sources but rather from accepting the need for change as your own, integrating exercise into your sense of self. And that can be learned."

Professor Teixeira's words set the stage for what you're going to do next. What follows is a list of twelve reasons to exercise. Some of them you'll probably read and think to yourself, *Yeah, I should probably try to exercise for that reason.* That's not the tepid reaction I'm going for! I want you to find the reason that inspires you to say, "*That* is what I care about." That's when you'll know you're on the right track. And once again, some of these reasons may seem familiar from the previous chapters.

Ultimately, you should exercise because you derive something positive from it—that's what's going to keep you going—so look for something that you feel will improve the quality of your life. Also be open to the idea that physical activity can give you pleasure. Really! You'll notice the pleasurable part of exercise when you pay attention to how you feel, especially *after* exercising, and you'll derive peace of mind from doing something you know is beneficial to your well-being.

THE WHY LIST: THIRTEEN REASONS TO EXERCISE (PICK AT LEAST ONE)

1. **You're worried about getting a debilitating and even deadly disease.** Let me propose this big one first. Exercise reduces the risk of just about every health problem, from stroke and cancer to diabetes and osteoporosis. The evidence that exercise helps to guard against cardiovascular disease, in particular, is very strong (you have half the risk of developing heart disease if you exercise), and researchers now believe that it offers protection in ways previously not known. When I asked an old classmate of mine who does research in this area, Michael J. Joyner, MD, a professor of anesthesiology at the Mayo Clinic, for an update, he said, "The ways

exercise protects your heart go beyond traditional risk factors such as blood pressure and cholesterol. We now also know that it reduces the type of inflammation that triggers heart disease, and dramatically improves the function of the lining of the blood vessels so that blood flows more easily to the heart."

Exercise is also a potent weapon in fighting type 2 diabetes, which is becoming epidemic in the United States. According to the National Institutes of Health, a healthy diet and exercise program can reduce your risk of type 2 diabetes by 58 percent. If you have a family history of diabetes, heart disease, or any of the other diseases physical activity helps prevent, you've got your reason to exercise right here.

2. **You want to not just lose weight but also avoid regaining it.** This is a given, but I wanted to list it as a reason anyway. As I will expand upon in chapter 6, people who maintain their weight loss work out regularly. They don't just exercise until they take off the pounds, then go back to sitting in a chair sixteen hours a day. If you really, really want to have a thinner, healthier body, there is no way around being physically active.

3. **You want to look better.** This doesn't mean that your motivation for exercising should be that you one day hope to appear in the Victoria's Secret catalog or on the cover of *Men's Fitness* magazine. It's important to be realistic and take your natural body type into account. That said, there is nothing wrong with wanting to look your best. It's a perfectly legitimate reason for exercising, as long as you keep in mind the limits of your own body and the limits of exercise to change it. Consider, too, that exercise doesn't help you look better just by reducing your weight; it also firms the body, improves posture, and gives the skin a glow.

4. **You feel grumpy, constantly annoyed, and sapped of energy.** Researchers at the Sacramento Veterans Administration Medical Center looked into this one and found that just one session of exercise—and it doesn't even have to be vigorous

exercise—can put you in a better mood for at least three to four hours. Sometimes the mood boost can last a whole twenty-four hours. People constantly tell me, "I just want to feel better." If you exercise regularly, you will. I haven't met anyone who wasn't eventually more energetic, less easily irritated, and calmer after working physical activity into his or her life.

5. **You're depressed.** It is a well-known fact that exercise helps lower depression, sometimes as effectively as antidepressant medications. Many psychologists even use it as part of the treatment for depression.

6. **You take too many sick days.** If you're looking for a way to reduce colds and upper respiratory infections, a good fitness program is it. Regular exercisers are 50 percent less likely to call in sick.

7. **You have muscle and joint pain.** The right kind of exercise (see page 276) can reduce the pain of osteoarthritis and rheumatoid arthritis by strengthening the muscles around damaged joints.

8. **You have a bad back.** Once upon a time, people with bad backs were urged to avoid physical activity altogether. But that practice went out the window a long time ago. In most cases, the best thing you can do for a bad back is move. Recognize your limits, of course, and work with your doctor and/or physical therapist to get moving again.

9. **You don't sleep well.** Even though exercise is energizing, it also wears you out. It's a paradox, I know, but take my word for it: Eventually you'll feel more vibrant during the day and sleep better at night.

10. **You want to slow the effects of aging.** Exercise is one of—if not *the*—most effective ways to fight aging. Loss of muscle and bone, two of the hallmarks of aging, are drastically reduced by exercise, and regular workouts also improve circulation, helping to prevent lines and wrinkles in the skin. Most important, exercise helps

reduce inflammation and causes other biochemical changes in the body that help stave off age-related diseases.

11. **You're concerned about staying mentally sharp.** Physical activity seems to have a protective effect against dementia, and helps improve memory and other cognitive functions. One Harvard University researcher has even referred to exercise as "Miracle-Gro for the brain."

MORE EXERCISE, LESS INFLAMMATION

There's a new buzzword in medical research these days. Perhaps you've heard of it: inflammation. Inflammation has been implicated in countless conditions, including heart disease, cancer, Parkinson's disease, Alzheimer's disease, and autoimmune diseases such as rheumatoid arthritis and lupus. When triggered by some kind of injury or infection, inflammation helps the body heal by promoting more immune activity in the affected area. But chronic, low-grade inflammation actually worsens unhealthful conditions, doing more harm than good.

Cardiovascular experts now believe that inflammation may play a significant role in heart disease. Certain factors, including smoking, high blood pressure, unfavorable blood lipids, and infections, can cause a release of chemicals that initiate the inflammatory process. That can contribute to the formation of plaque on the artery walls as well as the formation of blood clots. There is also some evidence to suggest that chronic inflammation—which can be a side effect of obesity, among other things—can lead to DNA mutations and, ultimately, the development of cancer.

One reason that exercise may have so many disease-fighting benefits is because it reduces the levels of proteins called pro-inflammatory cytokines as well as levels of another inflammatory protein, C-reactive protein. Exercise also seems to increase levels of an *anti*-inflammatory form of cytokines. In a roundabout way, it may also help by decreasing body fat and building muscle: Body fat actually produces *pro*-inflammatory cytokines that cause inflammation. Think about that next time you work out. You're knocking out inflammation with a one-two punch.

12. **You have asthma.** It may seem counterintuitive that the huffing and puffing of exercise can reduce asthma symptoms, but research shows that it's true. Physically active people with asthma also have fewer emergency room visits.

13. **You care about your kids.** When you care about yourself—and exercising is a sign that you do care about yourself—you are doing your kids a favor by setting a good example. Kids emulate their parents' behavior. If you're active, there's a better chance that your kids will be active, too. Plus, you'll also be doing your kids a favor if you stay healthy (see reason number 1) and are pleasant to live with (see reason number 4).

FIT DAD = FUN DAD

Peter Engwall is a well-conditioned and serious athlete. From half marathons and triathlons to 70.3-mile Ironman races, there isn't much the thirty-eight-year-old can't—or won't—do. Weighing in at a toned 190 pounds, the six-foot IT project manager drinks plenty of water, eats lots of fruits and vegetables, and keeps his body in tip-top shape with daily workouts. But Peter wasn't always the picture of health. In fact, just four years ago, he tipped the scales at 332 pounds and had trouble climbing up a flight of stairs.

What precipitated the transformation? "I wanted to enjoy life with my wife and son," explains Peter, whose son was four years old when his dad decided to start eating well and exercising. "I wanted to be the dad who played the game with his son instead of the dad on the bench. We used to go to the park, and I would see other dads chasing their kids around all morning long. I could barely keep up with my son and would have to sit to rest after running after him for just a minute or so. I also wanted to get in shape so I could go on the rides at Disneyland with my family. For several years, we had been asked by friends to go with them, and we always made up excuses why we couldn't. But deep down I knew the reason why we weren't going was because I couldn't fit on the rides, and there was no way I was going to be able to stand on my feet all day."

Peter decided it was time to make a change—a permanent one. He started *The Best Life Diet*'s eating plan shortly after the book was introduced in January 2007, then joined the

Add your own reasons here:

14. _____

_____

15. _____

_____

16. _____

_____

website: www.thebestlife.com. "Basically, I was overweight because I was lazy and I liked to eat," he says. "I knew, though, that I couldn't just go on a diet; I had to change my life." So Peter also joined the YMCA a couple of blocks from his office, and one day during his lunch break, he decided to actually go. "I got on the treadmill and just walked. The next thing I knew, thirty minutes had gone by, and I was completely wiped out. But it felt good. So I went back a couple of days later. Before I knew it, I *needed* to go; it was just feeling too good."

He continued increasing his activity and improving his diet, and in just ten months, Peter lost 140 pounds. Not only did he start to feel like a new man, but he finally became the type of father he wanted to be. "My son started calling me 'fun daddy.' We spent a lot more time playing: riding bikes, playing baseball, going to the park, and even jumping on a trampoline. We were active together."

Peter has kept the weight off for more than two and a half years, and he continues to improve his physical health by training for and participating in races and other athletic events. He credits his family with his continued commitment to his new lifestyle. "My family inspires me and motivates me every day to get up and get moving. They empower me. I want to strive to be the best I can be to set an example for my son that life is fun, and the easiest way to keep it fun is if you exercise and live a healthy lifestyle. Exercise is simply part of our lifestyle now, so no matter how we incorporate it, we get to it." Returning from his second family trip to Disneyland recently, Peter says, "We had an absolute blast!"

A PHOTO AND A TURNING POINT

Her church buddies kept coaxing her to join them at the gym, but Terane Weatherly, then a forty-two-year-old single mother of three, always turned them down. She felt awkward exercising because of her size. Then one day at work she had a seizure and was rushed to the emergency room—but she was too heavy to fit into the tube-shaped MRI machine. "The technicians really tried to stuff me in, but I just couldn't fit," recalls Terane, a senior associate at an insurance company who lives in Connecticut, and a participant in the National Weight Control Registry. "I was able to eventually get an MRI using an open-style machine, but that was at a later date. I had to face facts that if it were something serious, that delay could have been fatal."

Terane finally took her friends up on their offer. She could go only twice a week—she wasn't comfortable leaving her thirteen-year-old twin boys for more than that, and her eighteen-year-old daughter was not really interested in babysitting. "A gym is a very intimidating place when you've never been into physical fitness and you are the largest person there," says Terane. "Fortunately, the people I went with were very supportive, and the people I met at the gym were also encouraging." Outside the gym, she began walking for twenty minutes on her lunch break and tacking on a one-mile walk on the weekends. Six months later, she'd lost about 12 pounds.

Despite her progress, Terane's enthusiasm for weight loss and fitness was starting to wane—until she saw a photo of herself taken about three months before she started going to the gym. "I thought I was looking real good that day, but when I saw the photo, I felt horrible," says Terane. "I was five-foot-three, 285 pounds, and huge. I said to myself that I'd better take this seriously, especially the diet part, which I hadn't addressed. I joined Weight Watchers with my sister and kept going to the gym twice a week and walking on my lunch break."

At the gym, she spent thirty minutes doing cardio on the treadmill or elliptical machine and about twenty minutes strength training. Her weekend walks stretched from one mile to two or three. Plus, she started doing the little things that add up: taking the stairs instead of the elevator and parking at the farthest end of the lot. Two and half years later, Terane had lost 150 pounds, and to this day she keeps her weight between 135 and 141 pounds. Her exercise regimen has remained the same.

As she lost pounds, Terane found that she gained energy. "When I was overweight, I was so tired I'd come home from work and just sit there in front of the TV," she recalls. "I'd ask the kids to hand me stuff because it was hard to pick it up myself. Now I hardly ever watch TV; we don't even have cable. And I can do everything myself. I run up and down the stairs to retrieve things without thinking about it, and it's a lot quicker than waiting around for my children," she laughs. One of the most satisfying payoffs is that Terane's children have adopted her healthy eating habits, and the one son who was overweight is now at a healthy weight. She also has a lot more energy to devote to her passion: volunteering for her church, which includes getting on the road to help at homeless shelters, attending church conferences, "and basically anything that my pastors need me to do now that I have enough strength, energy, and determination."

Terane's story illustrates the point that what causes someone to transform herself can be surprising and unexpected. It might be something as minor as seeing a photograph—or it could be something more profound, such as surviving a life-threatening illness or going through a divorce. Keep in mind, though, that what triggers a turnaround isn't always the same as what helps you sustain your new, healthy life. In Terane's case, it began with a health scare, and shortly after, it was the photo that kept her going. Then, as she started feeling more energized, that became her new source of motivation. In any case, this initial turning point will help you look at your life, your weight, and your priorities in a totally different light, and when it hits you, you'll know it.

NO EXCUSES! STOP GIVING YOURSELF AN OUT

You may already have a good sense of how resistant you are to exercise and how agreeable you are to change. If not, a great way to assess your readiness, resistance, and willingness is to interview yourself using a technique called the motivational interview. To uncover any resistance you might have about changing your exercise habits, turn to page 243. There you'll find the thirteen questions and some tips on interpreting your answers.

Even if you are ready and willing to change, it's also important to ask yourself if you are able. Many people don't think they are. *I have no time. I'm physically limited. I can't wake up early enough. I'm too tired after work. I only like the weight machines they have at the gym, and I can't afford a membership. It makes me hungry. It doesn't make me skinny.* There are a million and one excuses, and yet hoards of people—even people with crazy, busy schedules and people who live with chronic pain—manage to exercise.

Excuses allow you to continue living the way you are now without making any tough choices or doing any hard work. They're a convenience, a way of allowing yourself to feel better about not doing things that you know you should do—and, somewhere deep inside, actually want to do. In order to move forward, you have to institute a zero-tolerance policy on excuses. Don't stand for them in yourself any more than you would stand for them in other people.

The people who make no excuses and go on to become regular exercisers offer proof that the old cliché "Where there's a will, there's a way" is still as valid as ever. Sometimes getting beyond the things that you typically make excuses for just takes creative problem solving. Sometimes it involves asserting yourself with family members or bosses to get the "me" time you deserve. Sometimes it takes seeking out an expert who can put you on the right track so that you ease into exercise and don't hurt yourself or burn out. What it always takes is an open mind and honesty. Making excuses is tantamount to lying to yourself.

What follows are excuses I routinely hear from people who live a sedentary life—and why those excuses aren't valid. Many of the barriers to weight loss are *perceived* barriers; they're not real. As you'll see, there are practical solutions to almost everything, and when you feel motivated and have a positive attitude, you're going to be open to resolving any perceived problems that stand in your way.

YOUR EXCUSE: "I DON'T LIKE EXERCISE"

Earlier in this chapter, I talked about the different reasons people don't like exercise, including bad experiences with formal physical activity in their youth and just plain old aversion to sweat, strain, and even workout clothes. While I appreciate your honesty about exercise, I still see it as an excuse. How many people like brushing their teeth at night when they'd much rather just fall into bed? But we all do it because we don't like the feeling of unclean teeth and don't want to end up with an unattractive smile or, worse, with a dentist's drill in our mouths. You need to take the same approach to exercise and do it because you need to; being physically active is a proactive strategy.

But I'm not advocating that you just grin and bear it. What I'm advocating is that you find a way to make it less of a chore. Take a few minutes to think about this: Is there *any* form of movement that you enjoy or can tolerate? There are so many different ways to move your body, from the simplest—walking—to the more complex, such as dance. Jennifer Demuth, profiled on the following page, took her first Zumba class (a dance class set to Latin music) and went from "loathing exercise" to becoming so into Zumba that she now teaches it. Look back at question 5 in your motivational interview. If you listed even one type of activity that has worked for you in the past, or if there's something else that seems appealing, you owe it to yourself to give it a try. Deciding not to exercise because you don't like an activity that you tried in the past is like deciding to never read a book again because you don't like mysteries. There are so many different ways to move your body; keep looking until you find the one that fits.

Remember, too, that there are also ways to enhance your exercise experience so that even if you're engaged in a workout you're not crazy about, you may not notice it. Tracy Ring, who you read about earlier, loves music, so she loads up her iPod with songs that divert her attention from the fact that she's pounding the pavement in her running shoes. Many dedicated exercisers work out with a television in front of them—it's amazing how quickly time passes when you're engrossed in a good movie or a favorite show. Others use their workout time as meditation, a time to get away from it all and quiet their minds. For more social people, I'm a big proponent of pairing up with a friend, both for distraction and because you're less likely to disappoint someone who's expecting you to work out. Shaun Tympanick, whom you met in chapter 1, and his brother started playing racquetball together and became hooked; they don't even notice how hard they're working.

FROM EXERCISE HATER TO EXERCISE INSTRUCTOR

Anyone who's ever taken Jennifer Demuth's Zumba fitness class would be hard-pressed to imagine that the five-foot-six, toned, high-energy instructor was once 260 pounds and a couch clinger. She hardly ever moved. "I spent my entire twenties at over two hundred pounds," says Jennifer. "It's hard to pinpoint what led to my weight gain, but it was most likely a variety of factors, such as having divorced parents since I was a toddler and struggling with the emotional turmoil of going back and forth between the homes of my parents and stepparents; low self-esteem; mild depression; job stress; and two miscarriages." So many situations in Jennifer's life made her unhappy, and food was one thing she felt she could turn to for comfort. It tasted good and was always there for her. To lose weight, she had to change the way she thought about and used food. She also had to find other ways to reward herself and reduce stress. "For instance, after completing a big work project recently, I went out and bought myself a new shirt," says Jennifer. "Before, I might have gone out for ice cream instead."

No matter how much you enjoy a sport or exercise, in order to have a productive workout, there's going to be a little discomfort. Not pain—there should never be pain—just the discomfort that goes with exerting yourself. That's a sign that the physiological changes that improve your health and burn calories are taking place. There's even some evidence to suggest that people who exercise develop a higher tolerance for pain, which may be of value if you have any painful chronic conditions.

With physical activity, as with anything in life, when you hang in there, you reap the rewards. Don't forget the reason you are exercising and use that to keep you going, even if you don't (and are convinced you never will) like exercise.

The turning point for Jennifer came when she was diagnosed with gestational diabetes, a form of the disease that crops up during pregnancy and is often caused by being overweight. "It was a real wake-up call for me to get on the road to good health, since my life and the life of my unborn baby girl depended on it," she recalls. With the help of a dietitian, she got her blood sugar under control for the final trimester and gave birth to a healthy baby girl. Then she lost 40 pounds, hovering at 220 for a while. At a plateau, Jennifer nudged her weight loss back into gear by joining a gym and hiring a personal trainer for a couple of months, who gave her a cardio and strength training regimen. "Then I discovered Zumba—I was so happy to find an exercise that wasn't boring and that I actually liked; I never thought I'd like exercise," she says. A year later, she'd lost 60 more pounds and has held steady at 160 pounds for close to two years.

As an instructor, Jennifer has particular empathy for exercisers struggling with their weight, just as she had. "I just want to encourage them and let them know it's possible without bariatric surgery or some get-thin-quick scheme," she says. "Never in my life would I have predicted that one day I'd be a fitness instructor—and that I'd love it."

YOUR EXCUSE: "I DON'T HAVE TIME"

Who isn't juggling a lot? Work, family, housekeeping, grocery shopping, your house of worship, personal finances, caring for an elderly parent, and all the rest of life's demands. If that's your life, activities that you feel are unnecessary—or, worse, unnecessary *and* boring—aren't going to make it into your day planner. But don't you always make time for the important stuff? If you're not exercising, it's because you haven't made it a priority.

One thing you can learn from people who are successful is how to make the time. People who work exercise into their lives on a regular basis tend to have figured out how to be more efficient with their time. They do a lot of double duty. One client of mine uses her morning workout to plan her day, including what she's going to make her family for dinner. (Your body has to be in the pool, but your mind doesn't.) You can also use this time to figure out where you're wasting minutes that you can otherwise spend on exercise. Another client uses exercise as meditation, an hour after work to clear her thoughts; it's a lot healthier than coming home and having a drink. One of my favorite stories is about a guy I know who was so concerned about time constraints that he built a desk over his treadmill; he works while he walks.

Find a way to work activity into things you already do. If you're a stay-at-home parent who can't make it to the gym, get a jogger stroller and walk or run your kids to the park. If you have an active social life, you don't have to give up hanging out with friends; just meet at a place where you can walk or ride bikes. Think creatively. Get to bed earlier so that you can strength train before your kids get up. Trade babysitting with a friend who would like to get in a workout, too.

Don't let situations that aren't perfect defeat you. Sure, it's a bummer if you can't make the morning spinning class at your gym, but you can still get on the exercise bicycle in your home. Maybe you can't walk around your neighborhood after work because it's too dark, but you can squeeze in a twenty-minute walk on your lunch break

A DIABETES WAKE-UP CALL

For most of her life, forty-year old Michelle Fairless was lucky. She ate moderately and exercised only once in a while, but she was able to keep her weight at around 120 pounds. However, after the birth of her third child in 2000, Michelle's luck ran out. Struggling to care for three children under the age of ten, she had little time to pay attention to her own needs, and the numbers on the scale began to climb, topping out at 165 pounds. Still, it wasn't until she received a diagnosis of type 2 diabetes in 2004 that she realized she had to get serious about her health.

"Finding out I had a life-threatening disease made me realize that I had to put myself first," says Michelle. "Bottom line, if I wasn't healthy, I couldn't be the wife and mom that I needed to be. Plus, I would have robbed myself of a full, quality life." She vowed to make some changes.

Not too long after, Michelle saw one of my appearances on Oprah's show, and it got her thinking about becoming more active. The first thing she did was to start using a pedometer to track her activity. "It was a huge wake-up call as to how inactive I really was," she recalls. Michelle started looking for easy ways to sneak in more everyday activity. "When I took my girls to their soccer practices, for instance, I didn't just sit and watch, I walked the field the entire time they were playing. Whenever I found a spare half hour at home, I walked around a nearby lake, and I started doing sit-ups on a balance ball every night."

Michelle also made a decision not to waste what little free time she did have doing things she disliked, like going to a gym. Instead she focused on finding activities that were fun. "I joined a fitness group, and they introduced me to the most beautiful trails in my area that I never even knew existed," says Michelle. As she stepped up her exercise and adjusted her diet, she dropped 35 pounds and completely reversed her diabetes.

Six years later, with no sign of diabetes and her weight holding steady at 130 pounds, exercise is simply part of who she is. "I do mud runs, triathlons, half marathons, turkey trots—there's always something fun every month that I'm involved in to help keep me motivated. I look forward to doing something active every day, even when I'm on vacation."

or hike through the corridors of your local mall before heading home. Take a page from Michelle Fairless's playbook (see page 153). She has to take her daughters to soccer practice, but instead of sitting in the bleachers, she walks around the field. There's a solution staring you in the face, and if you're motivated and if being active is a priority for you, you're going to get it done. Bear in mind, too, that as you become more fit, your energy and enthusiasm will rise so that you get more done at a quicker pace. In a sense, by taking time to exercise, you'll create more time elsewhere.

Here's something else you should consider if time is a problem for you. There are higher-intensity workouts that give you good results with a minimal investment of time. More and more research is showing that vigorous interval training can give you the same results as three times the amount of moderate-intensity exercise. Many electronic exercise machines offer an interval training option on their intensity controls, but you don't have to be on a machine to do it. Interval training involves speeding up to almost a sprint for a brief period—anywhere from thirty seconds to two minutes—then slipping back down to a moderate speed for either an equal amount of time or longer. You keep repeating the pattern, ending with a few minutes to cool down. One Australian study found that women who worked up to twenty minutes of interval training on an exercise bike three times a week lost about five and a half pounds of body fat in fifteen weeks. Other studies have shown that interval training for fifteen minutes three times a week changes the body in ways that help protect against diabetes and heart disease.

YOUR EXCUSE: "I'M NOT SURE WHAT TO DO"

Kickboxing, step aerobics, yoga, Pilates, kayaking, swimming, cycling, Afro-Brazilian dance, hip-hop, pole dancing, Spinning, walking on the treadmill or at an outdoor track or on the beach—there are literally hundreds of ways to exercise, and while that can be reassuring (you're bound to find something you like), it can also be very overwhelming. The only way you are going to know what you like is to experiment. But also keep in mind that different workouts work your body in different ways. Any exercise that you do is admirable, but if you want to really see changes in your body, you need to do a combination of exercises. Not only different types of *aerobic* exercise, though. To achieve true fitness, you need a three-pronged approach to exercise that includes these three elements:

1. Cardio (aerobic) exercise—measured either in minutes per day (or week) or by steps per day

2. Strength training

3. Functional fitness exercises

These are the different types of structured exercise you should perform. But unstructured exercise is important, too. Taking the stairs instead of the elevator, parking far from your destination so that you get in a little walking, getting up to talk to work colleagues instead of sending emails, walking rather than driving to the store—all these little things contribute to your overall fitness. If that informal type of inactivity is all you feel that you can fit into your life, I suggest that you purchase a pedometer, a small device that counts your steps, and aim to log a few miles that way. Appendix 6 contains a complete twelve-week fitness plan, including recommendations for step counting.

That plan is based on the following guidelines. Here, specifically, is how much of each type of exercise you need, depending on your goal.

CARDIO EXERCISE (ALSO CALLED AEROBIC EXERCISE)

To Lose Weight or Maintain Weight Loss

If you've been confused by how much cardiovascular exercise you need to do for weight loss or weight maintenance, you're not alone. There are many different guidelines out there, and they keep changing. My recommendation to clients is based on two things:

what research tells us works best and what I've seen firsthand while working with a variety of different people.

My recommendation to you is this: Gradually work up to exercising aerobically for approximately 6 hours (360 to 375 minutes) a week at a moderately high intensity. (See the Perceived Exertion Scale, on pages 158–160, for a guide to what different intensities feel like. Moderately high intensity is an 8 on the scale.) At first, this may seem like a lot of exercise, especially when you consider how inactive most Americans are. But keep in mind that you can break up those 6 hours however you like and choose whatever kind of physical activity you enjoy. Cycling or walking for an hour six days a week would do it, or you could exercise on an elliptical trainer or swim for 75 minutes five days a week. Doing a combination of activities throughout the week is another option—and a good one, as cross-training gives you the opportunity to build up different muscles and makes it less likely that you'll sustain any overuse injuries.

One area where my recommendation varies from some of the other ones out there is that I suggest that you always try to exercise at a *moderately high* pace. And here's why: Exercising hard dulls the appetite and keeps your eating in check. When you work out at a vigorous intensity, you just don't feel like eating after you're done and sometimes for hours afterward, making it less likely that you'll eat back the calories you just burned. Slower exercise, on the other hand, tends to stimulate the appetite, which can get you into trouble if you're trying to put the brakes on your eating.

If the moderately high pace I'm suggesting is too difficult for you, remember, this is a level of exercise you should work up to over several weeks. During that time, you can simply exercise longer and slightly relax the pace. You might, for instance, walk at a pace of 6 or 7 on the Perceived Exertion Scale, but for 1¼ hours instead of an hour. Another way to get all the exercise you need for losing or maintaining weight is to count steps: Ultimately, your goal should be 18,000 steps a day. That's about nine miles a day, which may sound like a lot, but you can accomplish this by going on formal walks and increasing your incidental walking. Not to mention, you're probably logging several thousand steps already in your normal day-to-day life without even realizing it.

Although you may not be ready to do 6 hours of cardio exercise weekly right off the bat, I encourage you to aim as high as you can when you first begin. Make your first goal 90 to 150 minutes per week, or at least 3,500 to 10,000 steps, the minimum amount for disease protection. If you're very overweight or have any medical conditions, check with your doctor before increasing activity.

To Protect Yourself from Heart Disease, Cancer, and Other Chronic Diseases

Get at least 2½ hours weekly of moderate intensity or 75 minutes of moderately high intensity exercise. Or do a combination of the two (for instance, 75 minutes of moderate and 38 minutes of moderately high intensity each week). Ideally, try to spread it out over five or six days a week. If you're currently not exercising, start with moderate intensity and bump it up to moderately high intensity only after a month or so, and if your doctor okays it. Alternatively, you can make sure that you take 10,000 to 14,000 steps a day.

Of course, if you can do more, great. For even greater protection against chronic diseases and to further improve fitness, get 5 hours a week of moderate-intensity aerobic exercise (or 150 minutes of moderately high intensity) spread out over most days of the week. Or, again, do a combo of moderately high and moderate intensity.

STRENGTH TRAINING EXERCISES (FREE WEIGHTS OR MACHINES)

For Both Health and Weight Loss or Maintenance

These guidelines for strength training also help the body beat back the effects of aging. Do a minimum of six different strength-training exercises that work the major muscle groups: abdomen, back, arms (biceps, triceps), shoulders, and legs (quads, hamstrings, calves). For each exercise, do at least two sets, eight to ten reps per set, at least two days a week—three days is even better. Begin with weights that are challenging but not so heavy that it's impossible to complete the eighth rep or they force you to compromise your form. I'd like to see you work up to eight or more strength-training exercises if you can. Ideally, three sets each (same number of reps), two or three times a week. You'll find more specifics on strength training in appendix 6, and for even more details, check out my previous books *Total Body Makeover* and *Get with the Program!* or visit www.thebestlife.com.

FUNCTIONAL FITNESS EXERCISES

For Both Health and Weight Loss or Maintenance

Being "functionally fit" is having the strength and agility to get through daily life with ease. Functional fitness also makes the other types of exercise you do easier and helps protect you against injury. The exercises that improve functional fitness are primarily stretches, crunches, and other resistance exercises (such as arm and leg raises and trunk curls) that you do with or without weights. As a group, they increase your core strength, flexibility, balance, and coordination. Ideally, you'd do functional fitness exercises every day. If that's impossible, do what you can. You can read more about functional fitness exercises in appendix 6 and on www.thebestlife.com.

THE PERCEIVED EXERTION SCALE

To bring about important changes in your body—changes that benefit your heart, your lungs, and the healthy functioning of just about every other part of your body—you need to exert some effort. The Perceived Exertion Scale helps you determine just how much effort you're exerting and whether it's enough to precipitate the changes you want. There are also formulas for figuring out how intensely you're exercising that rely on measuring your heart rate. Those are especially helpful for people who have specific heart problems.

However, I find that the Perceived Exertion Scale is easier to use and more accurate for the average person. This tool gauges how exercise feels to you, on a scale of 0 to 10. Using your breathing to gauge how much effort you're putting into your workout (you breathe harder as your exercise intensity increases because your body needs more oxygen to fuel your muscles), you ask yourself how hard you're working. That's your level of perceived exertion.

The optimum level of exertion is a 7 or 8. It may take a while for you to work up to this intensity—or to maintain it for any length of time—but it will come. If you can't hit that pace right off the bat, start at a lower level of exertion and try to exercise at a 7 for a minute or two before moving back to your more comfortable pace. Build on that, adding a minute each week (more frequently if you're able) so that you eventually work up to a whole workout at level 7 or 8.

0 This is the way you feel at rest. There is no fatigue, and your breathing is not elevated.

1 This is how you'd feel while working at your desk or reading. There is no fatigue, and your breathing is normal.

2 This is what you'd feel like when you're getting dressed. There is little or no feeling of fatigue, and your breathing is still normal.

3 This is how you'd feel while walking slowly across the room inside. You may feel a little fatigued, and you may be aware of your breathing, but it is still slow and natural. You also might feel this way in the beginning of an exercise session.

4 This is the way you'd feel if you were walking slowly outside. There is a slight feeling of fatigue, and your breathing is slightly elevated but comfortable. You should experience this level during the initial stages of your warm-up.

5 This is how you'd feel while walking somewhere at a normal pace. You're aware of your breathing, which is now deeper, and there is a slight feeling of fatigue. You should experience this level at the end of your warm-up.

6 This is similar to how you'd feel if you were hurrying to an appointment for which you were late. There is a feeling of fatigue, but you know you can maintain this level of exertion. Your breathing is deep, and you're aware of it. This is how you should feel as you transition from warm-up to your regular exercise session.

7   This is how you'd feel when you are exercising at moderate to moderately high intensity. There's a feeling of fatigue, but you're sure you can maintain this level for the rest of your exercise session. Your breathing is deep, and you're aware of it. You could carry on a conversation but would probably choose not to do so. You should try to maintain this level during your workouts.

8   This is how you should feel when you're exercising vigorously at moderately high intensity. You're feeling fatigued, and if you asked yourself if you could continue for the remainder of your exercise session, your answer would be that you think you could but you're not sure. You're on the edge, but you can maintain the pace, at least for a fairly good while. Your breathing is very deep, and though you could still carry on a conversation, you don't feel like it. You should try to exercise at this level only after you're feeling comfortable enough at level 7. Many people see rapid results at this level.

9   This is what you'd feel like if you were exercising very, very vigorously. You'd definitely feel fatigued, and you probably wouldn't be able to maintain this high-intensity level for very long. Your breathing is very labored, and it would be very difficult to carry on a conversation. If you're doing interval training, you may hit this level for short periods of time, but it's not a level that you need to or can stay at for a lengthy duration.

10   This level is all-out exercise, so difficult that you couldn't maintain it for very long. Hence, there's no benefit to it.

YOUR EXCUSE: "I'LL GET HURT"

If you haven't exercised much (or at all) in the past few years, perhaps you've talked yourself into the idea that you're too out of shape to exercise. One jog in the park, and you're sure to wind up sitting in the emergency room waiting for an ankle X-ray. Although you may be slightly more vulnerable to injury if you haven't taxed your body for a while, the threat of injury is very, very small. Most exercisers don't get injured, and a U.S. Centers for Disease Control (CDC) study of approximately six thousand men and women ages twenty-five to eighty confirms it: Over the course of a year, just a quarter developed any type of injury, and most of those injuries occurred while playing sports, not from walking or going to the gym. (Still, it's a good idea to get the green light from your doctor before beginning any exercise program.)

To my way of thinking, fear of injury isn't a valid excuse, and you need to see it for what it is: justification for not taking care of yourself. Any judge would throw that one right out of court. A good fitness option for many people is walking. It has a very, very low injury rate. Invest in a pedometer and follow the step-counting guidelines in the appendix.

YOUR EXCUSE: "I'VE SUFFERED AN INJURY"

An injury—whether it's lingering or newly acquired, exercise related or not—can seem like the perfect get-out-of-gym-free card. It seems only logical to abstain from any activity that might aggravate your bum ankle, cause your sore shoulder to swell up, or tweak an already tight muscle in your back. Years ago, you would have had your doctor on your side: Experts used to recommend bed rest or at least sitting it out until an injury fully healed. But while rest is still recommended, it's usually for a much shorter period of time (sometimes as little as a day or two, depending on the specific injury). Instead, a gradual return to activity has now become part of the recovery process for most injuries.

We now know that movement is essential to healing. For one thing, it increases blood flow to the injured area, bringing nutrients that help speed recovery. It also strengthens the surrounding muscles, taking pressure off the injured area, which allows it to heal more quickly and reduces the chances of reinjury. Staying active while injured also helps you maintain flexibility and range of motion, which are important to ensure full healing—if you don't have full range of motion or flexibility, you may heal only 80 percent or 90 percent. Plus, it will allow you to return to your full workouts more quickly. If you've stayed off your feet while nursing your injury, you'll lose strength, endurance, and flexibility, which will make it even harder for you to get back to where you left off.

This isn't to say that you should simply shake it off and get back out there if you're really hurt. And I'm definitely not recommending that you exercise through pain. See your doctor and let him or her guide you back into action. If your physician says that you're ready to jump back in (or get started), perhaps at a reduced level, but you feel resistant, this is a good time to check in to see what you're really feeling. Is it physical pain? Or are you procrastinating for some other reason? If there is no physical barrier preventing you from exercising, then there's obviously a psychological one, and you need to own up to it and explore the reason behind it.

If your injury truly is lingering, there are still ways to get in some form of activity, and, for the reasons I described above, it's in your best interest to do so. Think outside the box. If, for instance, you have an injury that affects your leg (shin splints, plantar fasciitis, or tendonitis of the knee or ankle, to name a few), you can do an arm-focused workout, such as using an upper body ergometer (basically, a bicycle for your arms) for cardio exercise, and perform upper body strength training exercises (such as biceps curls, chest presses, seated rows). You may even be able to participate in low-impact, non-weight-bearing aerobic exercise, such as swimming or walking in the water, which will give you a cardio challenge without putting stress on the injured area. If you're nursing an upper body injury (like a rotator cuff tear, tennis elbow, or even neck or back pain), you can do lower body resistance exercises (squats and lunges without weights) for your strength, and try an upright or recumbent stationary bike or elliptical trainer for your cardio workout. (Elliptical trainers come in both recumbent and upright versions. My favorite models are from Octane Fitness, www.octanefitness.com.) Runners who are injured usually do well when they switch to walking up a steep grade. It's still a vigorous form of exercise, but without the pounding.

As you return to exercise after an injury, it's also a good idea to ice the sore spot after you've finished working out. The body heats up with exercise, and as I noted earlier, that helps increase blood flow to the injured area. But heat also increases inflammation, and that can exacerbate the injury. Icing the area for ten to twenty minutes provides the best of both worlds: the heat-induced increase in circulation and all the nutrients it brings to the area from the exercise, plus the curtailing of inflammation from the ice. After you remove the ice, the blood rushes back in, once again bathing the area in healing nutrients.

Finally, make sure that you're able to distinguish a real injury from a little soreness or discomfort. It's completely normal to have minor generalized aches and pains in your muscles and joints after a workout or an activity in which you've exerted yourself (helping a friend move or doing yard work, for instance). An injury feels different, causing severe pain that's localized in one area of your body.

YOUR EXCUSE: "I HAVE A CONDITION THAT MAKES EXERCISE DANGEROUS OR PAINFUL"

When I think back on my bedridden great-grandmother, whom I wrote about in the introduction, I know that it would have been very difficult for her to exercise. She was that overweight. But I also know that obesity can be self-perpetuating and that it's important to do what you can until you're able to do more. While it's certainly true that excessive weight, arthritis, heart disease, diabetes, a neurological problem, or other chronic conditions can limit your exercise options, it's certainly *not* the case that no exercise is right for you. In fact, having a chronic condition typically makes exercise even more critical to your well-being. The symptoms of many health problems actually recede with exercise. (Of course, you should always check in with your doctor before beginning an exercise routine—and this is true for everyone, whether you're suffering from a chronic condition or you're perfectly healthy.)

No matter what your physical limitations, there's a way to get moving. Stop thinking of yourself as someone who "can't." Within reason, you can.

In appendix 6, you'll find guidelines for exercising with some of the most common chronic conditions, including arthritis, diabetes, fibromyalgia, heart disease, low back pain, and osteoporosis. These guidelines are meant to give you an idea of how to get moving, *but always work with your doctor* to flesh out an exercise program and make sure that you're not taking on too much. If you can afford a personal trainer who specializes in your condition, or your insurance will cover physical therapy, those are ideal ways to begin.

YOUR EXCUSE: "I HAVE NO PLACE TO EXERCISE"

If you're looking for a way out of exercise, logistical problems are not hard to find. You want to work out to a DVD, but your living room is too small. There are no good gyms or exercise studios in your area. You live in a neighborhood that is unsafe for walking. These are all legitimate complaints. However, if you are committed to getting active, you can find a way around these inconveniences.

It involves opening your mind to other options. You may prefer working out at home to a DVD, but if you can't reconfigure your furniture, it's not going to happen. (Yet also be aware that many DVD workouts don't require much space; you can do a lot within the narrow confines of an exercise mat.) So move on. Walk in your neighborhood, exercise in a park, or check out exercise classes at community centers, local Ys, and public parks. They may be more expensive than a DVD but are often reasonably priced and certainly a lot cheaper than private fitness studios. Public classes also tend to be low key. If you tend to feel uncomfortable in gyms that attract a lot of sleek bodies, you have another good reason to seek out the low-cost alternative.

If finding good exercise classes is your problem, but you can work out at home, then consider the DVD option. I have a *Total Body Makeover* DVD that is right for every level of fitness, and I am the virtual trainer on two EA Sports Active video games that you can use on the Nintendo Wii. But, of course, there are hundreds of at-home DVDs and virtual trainers out there. It is so easy to find good exercise instruction these days. You can even search for free yoga or Pilates podcasts on the Internet, which you can download to your phone. Access a few of them, and no matter where you go—on vacation for a week, to spend a weekend at your in-laws—you'll always have a workout on hand.

Living in a neighborhood where you don't feel safe exercising outdoors is definitely a challenge. And if you feel that way, you're not alone. A 2009 Gallup poll found that 42 percent of people without easy access to a safe place to exercise reported getting no exercise whatsoever. Interestingly, 30 percent of people who *did* have easy access to a safe place also got no exercise, so it's not just the police reports that stop people.

So let's think through some solutions. Could you drive or take public transportation to a nice park, better neighborhood, or school or university track? What about the neighborhood where you work? Could you exercise during your lunch break or arrive early or leave late so that you could take advantage of the area? Talk to your colleagues at work about joining you; some companies will even help you bring in an exercise instructor. And how about a mall? Malls are great places to walk and are the perfect option for anyone when the weather is inclement.

The point is, you do have options. Make the effort to seek them out.

KEEPING AN EXERCISE LOG HELPS

There's a reason that many people keep diaries, and it's not just because they want to preserve a record of their days for posterity. The physical act of writing lets you reflect on your actions (and, depending on what you're recording, often your feelings and ideas, too). An exercise log works in much the same way as a diary, which is why I recommend that you keep one. It also helps you stay honest. It's easy to "forget" the fact that you left the gym before doing any strength training, and harder to ignore it if you have to write it down. What's more, it's very motivating to see your progress in print.

The Lifestyle Log in appendix 1 will get you started. It's a comprehensive log that allows you to jot down all of the bouts of physical activity you engage in above and beyond walking around your house, office, grocery store, or other low-intensity activities of daily living. It also has room for other information that can help you pinpoint barriers that might get in the way of accomplishing your fitness goals. For instance, there is a "Sleep" column that allows you to note how many hours you sleep per night. If you find that you're frequently too tired to exercise, seeing your nocturnal habits in black and white might clue you in as to why. This log also has a "Food and Drink" column. While you don't have to fill in everything you eat, it will help you keep track of things like whether you're skipping meals or eating certain foods that lower your energy—either one can make your incentive to exercise wane.

Your exercise log serves a couple of other purposes. It's also a planner. At the beginning of the week, you'll write in exactly when and where you'll be exercising. This helps solve the "I don't have time" and the "I have no place to exercise" dilemmas; forced to fill in the blanks, you'll have to think of a solution. Granted, things don't always work out as planned. Changes happen, and it's actually to your benefit to be a little flexible when they do so that you don't get discouraged and give up on your routine altogether. But scheduling exercise in advance simply makes it much more likely that you'll do it.

Another advantage of keeping a log is that it lets you document some of the payoffs you're seeing from exercise. You might not even realize that your clothes are looser or that you're feeling and sleeping better until you have to think about it for your journal. Remember, weight loss isn't the only benefit that comes from physical activity. The log can help you keep that in mind.

For a more extensive log than the starter log found in the appendix, go to my website, www.thebestlife.com.

YOUR EXCUSE: "I DON'T SEE RESULTS"

Does it seem like working out just isn't working for you? Here are a couple of things to consider. First, while exercise helps with weight loss and, in most cases, is imperative for maintaining weight loss, exercise by itself generally doesn't trigger major weight loss for many people. You also have to cut calories.

When you begin exercising, your body plays a little bit of a trick on you. One way it responds to increased activity is by upping the amount of glycogen it stores in the muscles. The storage of glycogen, which is a type of fuel made from the carbohydrates you eat, requires approximately 2.5 to 3 grams of water per gram of glycogen. Therefore, as you become more active, you're going to be carrying around more water weight. More water is also stored in the bloodstream when you're active, adding even more water weight to your body. This physiological fact of life can disguise the real situation, which is that whatever exercise you're doing is probably causing you to lose body fat even though it's not showing up on the scale. That's why, in these early weeks of increased activity, I urge you to avoid the scale and gauge your progress by the way that your clothes fit. Most likely they will feel looser, and that is a good indication that the exercise is working. Ultimately, you'll stop putting on water weight, and actual body fat loss will begin to translate into a lower number on the scale.

What, though, are the results you are hoping for? That is something you should seriously consider. Is it simply the numbers on the scale that matter to you? My guess is that when you are exercising regularly, you actually experience a number of benefits, but that with lower weight as your primary goal, you're not noticing them. It may be that your arms and legs are stronger and more sculpted. Most regular exercisers have more energy, are less irritable, sleep better, and have brighter, healthier-looking skin. Moving your body also has payoffs—like better cholesterol, blood pressure, and blood sugar numbers—that are undetectable unless you've had a recent checkup from your doctor.

Another mark of progress is increased strength and endurance. Are you able to lift heavier weights than when you first began strength training? Can you last longer in your cardio workouts? Are you able to set the treadmill to a steeper slope or increase the resistance on other cardio machines? Can you walk twice as fast or as far as before? These are all signs that you are, in fact, getting results.

If you're at an unhealthy weight, having the numbers on the scale drop is important, and, truth be told, you may have to step up your game a little bit if nothing is happening. But don't drop exercise on the pretext that it's not getting you to your main goal, because you probably won't achieve that goal without it. Adjust your workouts and adjust your food intake to get your body into a calorie deficit and don't take for granted all the other extensive benefits of exercise.

YOUR EXCUSE: "I'M TOO TIRED"

Fatigue can become a vicious cycle. You're too tired to exercise, so you don't move much—which makes you even more tired. Plus, when you don't get physical activity, you miss out on its sleep-enhancing benefit, and that too can keep you in a state of low energy.

Have you asked yourself why you are so tired? Most people don't get enough sleep; maybe that's the reason. But fatigue is also a classic symptom of depression, something that Ann explored in detail in chapter 2. Mental stress is fatiguing too and can cause insomnia. Could either of these be sapping your energy? Being too tired to exercise is a sign that something is not right, whether it's an emotional issue you're sweeping under the rug, a physical condition that you need to see your doctor about, or an inability to effectively manage your life. If you are overwhelmed, your day packed to the rafters with too many responsibilities, something has got to give.

If you can nail down what is making you so tired and then take action to remedy it, you'll be on the road to becoming a regular exerciser. It's quite probable that the same thing that is keeping you from committing to healthy eating and exercise is also what's causing your fatigue. When you remove that factor, it's going to be easier for you to get into physical activity. But I wouldn't wait until then. As you're working out whatever issues you're dealing with, exercise can help give you the energy boost you need to confront anything, from a boss who has you working too many hours, to a spouse who doesn't pull his or her full weight, to the grief of losing someone meaningful to you. If you're tired because you're depressed, physical activity is also going to help lift your mood. If you're drained because you actually have a condition that makes you tired, such as fibromyalgia or chronic fatigue syndrome, exercise is still a necessity. In fact, it's one of the best things you can do to improve your symptoms and overall well-being.

It's also critical to realize that you're not always going to feel like exercising. Even the most psychologically and physically healthy people have days when they would just like to drop to the floor and take a nap! Yet many of them also push past the fatigue and get out there on their bikes or into the swimming pool because they know that within five minutes they're going to feel energized. Because, technically, that's what exercise does: It increases the production of hormones that put your body in a hyperalert state. One woman, a teacher, told me that she found herself practically nodding off in class after lunch. She decided to bring a pair of workout shoes to school and walk briskly three or four times around the school yard after she finished eating lunch. It worked just like a cup of coffee.

ACHIEVE YOUR GOALS

Throughout this chapter, I've prompted you to look at how motivated you are to exercise, to zero in on your own personal motivating factor or factors, and to own up to some of the excuses for not exercising that you may have made in the past. That's a lot to take in, but I hope that it has prepared you for what's to come next: setting your goals. To help you, we've provided a goal-setting worksheet for you in appendix 4, which requires you to get very specific about your aims and how you hope to accomplish them. For instance, instead of writing, "I need to spend more time at the gym," I want you to plot out exactly when you'll go to the gym this week and how you'll overcome barriers to getting there. Or, instead of writing, "I need to start walking," you're going to figure out exactly when, where, and how this will occur. After you complete the worksheet, you're going to have a manageable, realistic plan in hand.

A few years ago, researchers at Columbia University in New York City and the University of Konstanz in Germany conducted a joint study looking at what helps people stick to exercise. They found that women who filled out a goal-setting worksheet *doubled* their weekly workout time compared to a similar group of women who did not use the technique.

The worksheet in the back of this book is based on the one used in that innovative study. To give you a sense of what your worksheet might look like, I filled out a sample one (also used to good effect in one of my previous books, *The Best Life Guide to Managing Diabetes and Pre-Diabetes*). In appendix 4, you'll find a blank sheet that you can fill out yourself. As you'll see in the chapters to come, this worksheet will also help you set goals in other areas of your life.

When you fill out the worksheet, stay specific and realistic. Start by using it to set a goal for the next twenty-four hours. Then repeat the exercise tomorrow, but this time, give yourself a two-week goal. If your life were a business, a worksheet like this would comprise your mission statement and strategic plan all in one. That is, you'd be ready to put theory into action. So don't wait. Fill out the one in the back of the book and make your plan a reality!

WHAT YOUR GOAL-SETTING WORKSHEET MIGHT LOOK LIKE

1. **What is my exercise goal?** Find a goal you know you can achieve; nothing overly ambitious. For instance: "getting thirty minutes of exercise in the morning."

2. **What is the most positive outcome of achieving this goal?** This is crucial. Think back to the earlier section when you thought about reasons to exercise and which one or ones resonated with you. If you can't visualize a positive outcome, it's going to be hard to keep up your motivation. Imagine and name a benefit. For instance: "Doing this regularly will get me in better shape and help me better manage my diabetes."

3. **What is the main obstacle standing in my way?** For example: "I don't have enough time to work out in the morning."

4. **How can I overcome the obstacle?** Give details, noting the "when" and "where" of the changes you're going to make to overcome the obstacle. For example: "In the morning, I can skip reading the newspaper at the kitchen table, which will give me twenty more minutes. Also, the night before, I can turn off the TV and get to bed an hour earlier—by ten—so I can wake up earlier and give myself another fifteen minutes in the morning."

5. **How do I prevent the obstacle from occurring in the first place?** Again, be precise. For example: "I could make ten o'clock my new bedtime, and from now on read the newspaper later in the day."

6. **How, specifically, should I achieve my exercise goal?** This means focusing on specifically when and where it will happen. For example: "Between six-thirty and seven in the morning, I'll exercise with a thirty-minute aerobics video in my living room and then take a shower."

STAYING MOTIVATED

Making excuses can be habit forming. When one excuse is plainly no longer legitimate, you come up with another one and then another one. It feeds on itself. On the other hand, overcoming excuse making is freeing. You can stop hemming and hawing and wasting energy trying to come up with reasons why you can't exercise. Instead you see things very clearly. You are an exerciser, it's part of your life, you (to borrow a phrase) just do it. It's like dinner, a part of your day, a ritual. When you reach this point, you don't even have to worry about staying motivated. You've become a different person. An active person.

5

TRANSFORMING YOUR BODY IMAGE

By Ann Kearney-Cooke

TAKE A SECOND TO think about your body: What springs to mind? Are your thoughts mostly positive, primarily negative, or somewhere in between? About half of us—56 percent of women and 43 percent of men—are dissatisfied with our overall appearance. I think it's safe to say that if you're reading this book, there's a good chance you're in that camp as well. Don't worry, we're going to help get you out of it.

Maybe you have a generally healthy body image but struggle a little. (Say you're fixated on one area, like your legs or your stomach.) Most people can pinpoint things they like about themselves—including their hair, face, and height—if they're asked to, but a large percentage still admit to feeling unhappy about their body—in particular, their abdomen and weight. In fact, according to research, an astounding 89 percent of people say they want to lose weight. Even in these cases, it's worth working to accept and even embrace your body. That's because your body image, or the mental representation you have of your body and the thoughts and feelings that go along with it, affects your self-esteem, which in turn influences every area of your life. Studies have linked low body image to anxiety, depression, sexual dysfunction, and eating disorders.

If your body image is lacking, you're more likely to feel unworthy of good things in your life. This pessimism may then affect relationships with friends, family, and co-workers, and it factors into everyday decisions, such as what you eat, how you dress, and where you go. In the end, your lack of confidence and the dissatisfaction you feel with yourself will prevent you from ever trying to repair your fundamental body image issues.

Fortunately, you have the ability to change. In this chapter, you're going to learn to start seeing your body from a new perspective, and if you have a poor body image, you're going to work on improving it. You might even discover that you're actually hanging on to these negative or bad feelings about your body—maybe because you fear you'll lose your motivation to slim down or get in shape if you become more comfortable and accepting of yourself. Or perhaps you've always made light of your weight and body image, insulting and hurting yourself before anyone else can. You might think it's easier when *you're* the one telling the fat jokes. It could even be that it's just more comfortable for you to live with these negative feelings. Holding on to a poor body image can be soothing, oddly enough—the belief that you're not attractive or not worthy feels familiar and safe. You might even derive a hidden sense of pleasure in living up (or down) to the expectations of overly critical parents or others that have been drilled into your head for years, or that you've heard time and time again from an emotionally abusive spouse. For many people, being fat simply becomes part of who they are. Learning to accept and love yourself requires letting go of this identity and creating a new one for yourself, and that can be very difficult.

But accepting and believing that you are worth it, that you do deserve happiness, and that your body is good and beautiful and strong are profound changes that only breed more happiness and confidence. When you feel good about yourself and your body, you'll want to take care of it, feed it healthy foods, exercise, and insist that the world treat you with respect. Feeling strong brings about changes in other areas of your life, too. You'll carry yourself with more confidence, which could help you advance in your career, strengthen your relationship with a significant other, make you a better parent, give you the courage to try new things and experiences—the list is really endless.

So it's time for you and your body to end the rivalry and join the same team, because you can't live a healthy, motivated life without feeling good about yourself and your body. Not to mention, if you don't learn to value yourself and your body, it becomes even easier to give in to the temptations to stop eating healthfully and exercising. The first step toward acceptance: letting go of negative versions of yourself and your body. Every time you catch yourself saying or thinking things like: *I will never be fit, I will never be attractive, I will never be sexy again, I can never stop overeating,* and so forth, replace them with body-positive mantras such as: *I can be attractive; I can be fit; people do overcome overeating, and I am going to be one of them.*

If you've struggled with your body image since you were a child, it's time to acknowledge that you can't change what was said about or done to your body in the past. However, you *are* in charge of how you treat, talk to, and relate to your body and how you allow others to do the same! And if your body image issues are more recent, you're going to figure out where they came from and learn how to turn things around.

BODY IMAGE BASICS

Body image might not get a lot of attention until the teen years. You often hear about middle school and high school as a formative time for body image issues. Girls struggle with eating disorders and the pressure to be thin, and young boys also deal with the stress of trying to fit in. Yet, by then, your body image has been developing for many years. Your view of yourself originates with the positive or negative reactions—words, nonverbal cues, and touch—of your parents. As a child, you internalized the ways that you were touched, talked about, and accepted or rejected by others throughout your development.

Marie Lewis, a thirty-five-year-old overweight woman, describes the impact that her parents had on her in the following way: "Being around my overly critical parents has left scars. From as early as I can remember, my mother and father told me I was fat and needed to lose weight. As a result, when I look at myself, I focus on what I don't like about my body. Instead of saying, 'I have lost over thirty pounds in the past year, and I am more fit now than when I was a teenager,' I say, 'You are fat and have huge thighs and a huge stomach.' It's as if my parents' harsh words from the past were branded into my brain. They leave me feeling hopeless and unmotivated."

Sometimes the criticisms from parents are more subtle. While your mother and father may not have been as blunt as Marie's, they may have still communicated their dissatisfaction with your body or looks by saying things like: "You're not going to eat that whole piece, are you?" or "You know you don't look good in blue; why don't you go change?" Or perhaps your parents never said anything—good or bad—about your body. Even still, they had a major effect on your body image; how they felt and talked about their own bodies shaped the way you see yours. If you grew up with a mother who was constantly putting herself down—"I look horrible in a bathing suit" or "I hate my arms"—it's almost inevitable that you'll inherit some of this negative thinking about your own body. Or maybe your mother was always on a diet. The message that sends is that thin is ideal and everything else is unacceptable. Ironically, it could even be that your parents did everything right: They were supportive and encouraging and were healthy role models themselves, but the pressure you put on yourself to live up to their example sent you in the opposite direction. This is what happened with Tracy Ring (whom you met in chapter 4), one of the Best Life challengers who was profiled on *The Oprah Winfrey Show*. Her parents lived a very active life and encouraged her to do the same. But this only backfired: Tracy ended up doing whatever she could to avoid exercise. Fortunately, she was able to work through it, and now she's participating in triathlons. She has completely turned her life around.

As you remember back to your childhood, also try to think of your friends or classmates and how they treated you; they may have also had a hand in how you feel about your body, as teasing or bullying during adolescence can lead to poor body image. Something as seemingly minor as being picked last for a team in gym class, not being asked to the prom, or being excluded by the popular clique can leave a mark, whether you're aware of it or not. And traumatic events such as sexual or physical abuse can have a profound and often devastating effect on body image, leaving the victim feeling dirty or ashamed.

All of these things form the basis of body image, but as you go through various stages of your life (school, career, marriage, family, and so on), it continues to change and evolve. This can be a good thing. For instance, if you've struggled with your body image as a child, you may have gained a healthier perspective as you grew into adulthood. I often see this with young women after they give birth. They develop a new respect for their body because they've turned their focus to what it can *do* (carry a baby, birth a baby, breastfeed), not just how it *looks*.

The countless images and messages we're exposed to on a daily basis throughout our lifetime also play a role in our body image. The media helps set a culture's standard of beauty. The ideals in our culture are so unrealistic that less than 5 percent of the population meet them. Research shows that twenty-five years ago, top models and beauty queens weighed only 8 percent less than the average woman; now they weigh at least 23 percent less. Unfortunately, many of the ideals that define beauty are computer generated: Blemishes are buffed out, legs are made longer or thinner, and any trace of fat is airbrushed away. Yet there's pressure to try to live up to these images, no matter how unrealistic or unhealthy they are.

Anne Becker, a Harvard anthropologist who had been studying life on Fiji since 1988, carried out a really interesting research project. On the small island in the Pacific Ocean, the fuller-figured woman was once the cultural ideal. In fact, there were essentially no cases of eating disorders prior to 1995. What happened in 1995 to change things, you might be wondering. That's when the island's only TV station started broadcasting American shows like *ER* and *Melrose Place*, which featured predominately thin actresses. Three years later, Becker found that 74 percent of girls felt they were "too fat or too big," and 11 percent reported that they'd practiced purging to control their weight.

Another factor that influences body image: how you're feeling in general. For instance, when something isn't going quite right in your life—a failing relationship, financial stress, the loss of a job—you may project this negative feeling onto your body. So instead of saying that something is wrong with your relationship, your finances, or your work, you say that something is wrong with your body. I see this problem with so many of my clients.

As you can see, body image is complicated: It's shaped by your history as well as your here and now. It's influenced by other people—your relationships from the past as well as the present ones—and by personal factors, from your mood and beliefs, to your body type and weight. And it's also affected by outside forces, like our culture. Taking the time to assess how you view your body, and why, is the first step to understanding and accepting yourself. Then you can begin to gradually chip away at the forces that

A CHEEKY RETORT

Forty-three-year-old Susan Burke was a member of a weight-loss group I led years ago. Her husband criticized her weight, especially the size of her butt. Genetically, she was wired to have a large butt; her mother and sister did, too. One day, we talked about the importance of teaching people how to talk about and treat your body regardless of your weight. This was one of the steps of developing a healthy body image. She went to her doctor that week for her yearly checkup, and he said, "Good for you! You have lost eighteen pounds, you have color in your cheeks, and your cholesterol level is down. Your workouts are really paying off. You look great."

Later that night, while looking at herself in the mirror, Susan said to herself, *He's right, I look fit and feel better than I did in my thirties.* Her husband came in and said, "What are you doing?" She told him about the good news and extensive praise from her doctor. Her husband replied, "What did he say about your ass?" She retorted, "He was busy—he didn't have time to talk about you!"

Susan shared with the group how great she felt when she responded to her husband's derisive comment. Her whole life, she had apologized for having a big butt—this was the first time she had stood up for her body. Instead of filling up on doughnuts in response to his remarks, she felt empowered. She went straight to bed and said to herself, *This is the last time I will put up with anyone putting my body down!*

have contributed to your poor body image. The exercises in this chapter, as well as the inspiring success stories, will help you get started on this journey.

Of all the factors that knock down (or build up) our body image, there are many that we can't control, such as how we were treated as a child by our parents or peers, our cultural ideals, and any traumatic events we may have suffered. Yet we're not completely powerless when it comes to body image barriers. The most common and most important obstacles, listed below (some of which you've read about briefly in chapter 2), are things that you *can* change and overcome—and I'll be offering practical advice on how to do it.

BARRIER: A NEGATIVE FOCUS

Do you spend too much time criticizing your body, focusing on the negative, and ignoring the positive? You may not even be aware of this negative self-talk, in which case you'll have to make an effort to notice how often you harbor negative thoughts about your body. Do you ever take the time to really look at your body—for example, when you get out of the shower or as you're undressing—or do you avoid the mirror at all costs because you are disgusted with your body? Does this self-loathing drain your energy and affect your relationships at work and at home? Try the following exercises once a week for the next few months and train yourself to look at your body in a more positive light by identifying your signature body strengths. You may be resistant to doing some of these exercises, but I encourage you to give them a try. They've been very effective for many of my clients.

Step 1: Perform the Mirror Exercise

Find a room in your house where you can stand in front of a mirror for fifteen minutes without being interrupted. Take off your clothes or leave on only your underwear and slowly look at your body as if you're seeing it for the very first time. Take a look at each body part in a loving and kind way. Look at your face and pay special attention to the parts of your face that you find the most attractive. Focus on these parts and admire them. Then look at the upper part of your body, including your arms, neck, and chest. Which parts of your upper body do you like? Focus on these parts and admire them. Now look at the middle section of your body, including your stomach, thighs, and buttocks. What do you like most about the middle section of your body? Focus on these things and admire them. Finally, look at the lower section of your body, including your legs, knees, and feet. What body parts do you like from the lower section of your body? Focus on them and admire their beauty.

Try to notice the beauty of different parts of your body the same way that you would focus on a loved one's body: shapely buttocks, full breasts, curvy hips, plump lips, and so on. Remind yourself that it's not only okay but motivating to appreciate your body as it is, even when you are in the process of trying to lose weight.

Step 2: Identify Your Signature Strengths

Now write down the parts of your body that you consider attractive. For each part, think about ways that you can enhance and nurture it so that you can come to embrace and appreciate it even more. Periodically, using this format, list as many signature strengths as you can think of in a notebook or journal.

EXAMPLE

Signature strength: *my muscular arms*
I can take care of them by: *continuing to weight train*
I can embrace them by: *wearing sleeveless dresses*

Signature strength: _____
I can take care of it/them by: _____
I can embrace it/them by: _____

If you are struggling to identify your signature strengths, ask those closest to you what they find most attractive about you. Although this may sound a little strange, people who really care about us enjoy pointing out our attractive features.

Step 3: Set Healthy Body Image Goals and Track Your Progress with an Activity Log

Learning to highlight and appreciate your strengths can make it easier to accept and work on your weaknesses. Still, changing your thinking won't be easy. The following exercise can help you gradually break some bad habits and transform how you see your body.

Here's how it works: Using the worksheet below (or your journal), write down a healthy body image goal you have for yourself. For instance, yours might be to eat healthfully and to feel good about your body. At the end of each day, write down the behaviors or things you did to help bring you closer to that goal. Also note where you fell short of this goal, and think of ways that you can deal with these slipups going forward in the "Negative Behaviors and Action Strategies" section.

Finally, score yourself from 0 percent to 100 percent, with 100 percent signifying that you have fully achieved your goal. After the first week, you might only be at 10 percent, but by continually engaging in body-positive behaviors, you will gradually move up to 60 percent and 80 percent, which means you are getting closer to accepting your body and taking care of yourself. Sticking with the example above, your Activity Log might look something like this:

GOAL: I want to eat healthfully and feel good about my body.

Body-Positive Behaviors

1. I woke up early and walked for forty-five minutes while listening to my favorite CD.

2. When I overate at lunch, instead of bingeing all day, I got back on track at the next meal.

3. I went out dancing with my coworkers after work, and I really enjoyed myself.

4. I taught my significant other how to touch my body in a more nurturing way.

Negative Behaviors and Action Strategies

1. I found myself criticizing my body while getting dressed for work. Next time I should visualize a stop sign, tell myself to stop, and replace the negative thoughts with positive affirmations such as, "My arms look great in this dress, and I'm glad that I've been strength training two times a week."

2. I got upset with my boss and turned to a bag of chips to calm myself down. Next time I can go for a walk in the parking lot instead of hitting the vending machine.

Score: 80 percent. Overall, this was a great day. I ate healthfully most of the time, participated in positive and motivating activities, and connected with my partner better. However, I did rely on food to get me through a stressful work situation, and I did catch myself putting my body down once, so I couldn't give myself top marks.

Now, it's your turn. Give it a shot using the Activity Log below.

GOAL: _____

Body-Positive Behaviors

1. _____

2. _____

3. _____

Negative Behaviors and Action Strategies

1. _____

2. _____

3. _____

Score: _____%

This exercise was a big help for one of my clients when he was tempted to go off track. In his Activity Log, twenty-eight-year-old Michael Miller described waking up depressed and unmotivated one Saturday morning. He wanted to sleep in, drink some beer, order pizza, and watch sports all day. However, because he had been working on his Activity Log the night before, he remembered action strategies that would bring him closer to his goals and make him feel better. So he got up, went to the YMCA, and worked out with weights and joined a pickup basketball game. Although he was tired afterward, he felt reenergized. He stopped and got some healthy Chinese food and visited his father to watch some football with him.

Every night before you go to bed, close your eyes and picture yourself engaging in body-positive behaviors the next day. For example, see yourself at the conference you'll be attending and then picture yourself swimming in the hotel pool before dinner. Setting this imaginary intention can help you to stick with your plan if someone or something interferes with your goals—for example, a favorite colleague wants to meet you for a drink during this time. Not only would you have to miss your planned swim, but you know that drinking before dinner often triggers overeating the rest of the night. Imagine yourself warmly and confidently telling your colleague that you can't have a drink but that you do want to sit next to her at dinner to catch up. Then see yourself swimming in the pool and engaging in a delightful conversation with your colleague at dinner.

BARRIER: A LACK OF EMPATHY FOR YOUR BODY

No one is immune to the bony-is-beautiful message that we're bombarded with day in and day out. Even if your parents worked hard to instill in you a strong sense of self-worth while you were growing up or you consider yourself a pretty well-adjusted adult, you can't help but be affected by the near-skeletal models and sculpted celebs who are on the covers of fashion magazines, billboards, TV programs, and commercials. It doesn't matter if you're actively taking in these messages or just passively absorbing them—either way, they can be downright toxic.

That's because it's human nature to compare yourself to the ideal, regardless of how unrealistic it might be. According to the widely accepted psychological premise called the social comparison theory, individuals appraise others to make judgments about themselves. You may find yourself comparing yourself to others of the same age, height, and so on in order to evaluate how you feel about yourself and your own body. Almost everyone is likely to have a discrepancy between their actual appearance and the ideal appearance to some extent, but when you're comparing yourself to today's dangerously thin ideals of beauty, that gap only widens, particularly for those who are overweight or obese.

The fact is that most of us will never get down to a size 4—let alone the model-thin sizes of 0 or the more absurd 00, the size *below* size 0—no matter how much we work out or how healthfully we eat. Very few people are genetically wired to maintain that weight or size, and many models who *do* reach this size rely on dangerous diet or exercise tactics, or even drugs, to get and stay there. Yet we still hold ourselves up to these ideals and feel disappointed when we fail to reach them. You might feel as though something is wrong with you or that you don't measure up, and are ashamed and self-conscious about your shape and weight. Perhaps you become angry with your body for "falling short," and engage in those aforementioned risky dieting and exercise regimes. Instead of appreciating everything your body has been through and continues to do for you, you hate it, put it down, ignore its signals and cues, and become increasingly disconnected from it. If this sounds familiar, then you'll have to work on changing your perspective, because you'll never be successful with weight loss until you can move from anger and shame (a state of *disconnection*) to empathy (a state of *connection*).

Staring at überskinny starlets is only part of the problem. This thin-is-in thinking permeates our society, so the further you are from the ideal, the less accepted you may feel or actually be. Whether you've been overweight since childhood or your struggles with weight began during adulthood, you've probably experienced fat prejudice. You may have been teased, harassed, or bullied as a child because of your weight. You may have been put down by your parents or other authority figures, or experienced size discrimination as an adult. Over time, it's natural to internalize weight bias and buy into weight-based stereotypes—for instance, that obese people are lazier than thin people—which increases your vulnerability to depression, anxiety, poor body image, and lower self-esteem. Regardless of your weight or shape, you deserve to be treated with respect.

Challenging negative self-talk and developing empathy toward your body is an important step toward a healthy body image. In the following exercise, you'll pick a body part that you typically dislike or criticize (such as your hips, butt, or thighs) and imagine that you're that part. In essence, you'll be forced to defend yourself as the "problem" part. This will help you understand how negative words and actions affect your body. To begin, name the body part you dislike most, then write down the answers to the questions below from the perspective of that body part.

1. What is the body part you are most dissatisfied with?

_____

2. How do you treat this part?

_____

3. What does this part need from you now?

_____

Mary Lopez, a thirty-six-year-old working woman who hated her belly, did this exercise. She wrote, "My stomach told me to stop putting it down, squeezing it into clothes that are too tight, and eating out of control at night. My belly said, 'I am getting tired of you criticizing me and putting me down. You barely eat until dinner, when you stuff me with too much food and diet soda. I feel sick and neglected. I want you to stop bingeing at night, drink water, and become more active.'"

Most people with body image issues have several parts they dislike; practice this exercise with all of those parts. You may be surprised by how much your body has to say. And you may also be disappointed in yourself at how you treat your body, particularly the parts you don't like. Hopefully, this exercise will help you realize that it's time to start listening to your body and responding to it in a loving, kind way.

BARRIER: AN UNREALISTIC WEIGHT GOAL

Although many body factors can contribute to a negative body image (scars, freckles, and cellulite, to name just a few), weight is certainly one of the most common triggers—if not *the* most common. For those with weight-related concerns, the key to developing a positive body image as you work on slimming down is to set a realistic weight goal. Instead of taking into account genetic predisposition, body shape, and bone structure to determine an appropriate weight loss goal (as well as a realistic time frame to meet this goal), many people aim to get back down to the weight they were in their twenties or the number they were before they married or had kids. But this number may not be possible or even healthy for many people. The bottom line: If you aim for a weight that you have little chance of ever achieving, you'll most likely end up with feelings of failure and disappointment, which will result in an even poorer body image. Researchers have found that people who begin weight loss with unrealistically high expectations as well as those with an accepting attitude ("I'll be happy with minimal weight loss") lose the least amount of weight. The people who achieved the greatest loss were those who had moderate expectations.

Smaller, attainable goals can help you stay motivated as you try to lose weight. For instance, many successful individuals begin with a goal of shedding 5 percent to 10 percent of their weight: So, if you weigh 180 pounds, a reachable target would be to lose 18 pounds. After they lose that weight, they go into a maintenance phase for a period of time and then strive to lose an additional 5 percent to 10 percent of their body weight. You can continue this process until you reach your end goal or your BMI falls into the normal category. (See appendix 2 for more on BMI.)

In addition to setting a goal that you can reach, you also have to allow yourself a reasonable amount of time to get there. Weight loss experts agree that for most people, a loss of 1 to 2 pounds a week is healthiest. That means, if you need to lose 18 pounds, prepare to embark on at least a three-month program. Losing weight slowly means that you have time to develop healthy new behaviors, such as eating more nutritiously and exercising more. Remember, diets don't work; changing *behaviors* does! Set short-term goals so that you stay motivated. And don't forget to reward yourself when you hit them. For example, circle the date on your calendar every day that you eat healthfully and exercise. Once you have ten circles, treat yourself to a new belt, manicure, massage, or the like.

Finally, no matter what goal weight you choose, you have to be willing to make reaching it a priority. I have found that most people will need at least an hour and a half a day to work on their weight loss goal: allotting time to exercise (including travel to and from the gym), to meditate and relax, and to eat healthfully (cutting vegetables, grocery shopping, and so on).

The exercise below allows you to examine how you use your time and can help you free up some of your day for exercise or healthy eating. It identifies the demands on your time and the percentage of each day you spend on various activities. The pie chart on the left represents a typical day for a working man or woman. It shows eight hours devoted to work; eight hours for sleep; four hours for carpooling, television, helping

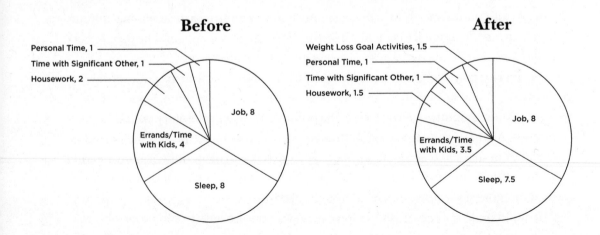

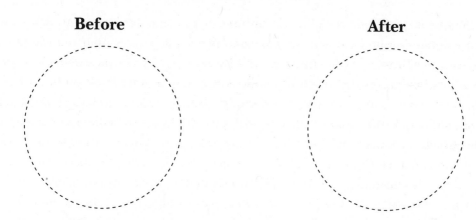

Before　　　　　　　　　　　　**After**

kids with homework, and hanging out; two hours for taking care of the house, laundry, and other chores; one hour to be with your significant other; and one hour for personal time, such as reading, checking email, or talking to friends. The second pie chart revises the time allocation to reflect weight loss goals as a priority.

Now it's your turn. Use the "before" pie chart above to clarify the current demands on your time, then use the "after" pie chart to redistribute your time so that you make weight loss a priority. Ask yourself how you can put aside about an hour and a half each day to allow enough time to meet your weight loss goals. Your body image and overall health are invaluable, so you should be willing to invest the necessary time and money into improving both, no matter how long that takes.

BARRIER: AN AVERSION TO SOCIAL SITUATIONS

The process of losing weight is difficult, but the challenges of staying overweight are often even tougher. Aside from the obvious health consequences involved with carrying around too much weight (an increased risk for heart disease, stroke, diabetes, some cancers, depression, and more), you also must deal with the social effects: being stared at or teased, feeling isolated from others, having to miss out on experiences because you're not in good enough shape, and dealing with shame.

Shame is such a powerful emotion, one that arises when we're disappointed about who we are, how we look, or our basic nature. Regret or guilt, on the other hand, is a feeling that results from a certain action or mistake we may have made. Shame related to our body or self can affect every area of our lives, from how we eat to how we interact with the world. For instance, many people who feel overwhelmed, out of control, and ashamed by their weight, their behavior, or their inability to slim down avoid social situations for fear that they may be "found out" as the flawed person they believe they are. They're afraid of rejection or derogatory comments from others. They don't want anyone to see how much weight they've gained or how fat they are or even when they eat. So they continue to withdraw. They don't go to their friend's baby shower or meet coworkers for dinner. They skip their high school reunion or family vacation. They steer clear of the gym. They isolate themselves because it feels safe.

But this only perpetuates the problem. When you avoid going out with others, you may instead engage in addictive behaviors to numb your feelings of shame and lonliness. The relief gained through overeating is only temporary, and the subsequent feelings of remorse compound the deep feelings of shame within.

The solution is to face your fears head-on by pushing yourself to engage with others socially. You'll benefit enormously from the fitness instructor's encouragement at the gym, the camaraderie of walking the neighborhood with friends, and the great time sharing stories with coworkers at an after-work get-together. The simple fact is that we cannot heal when we hide from ourselves or from others.

If these types of interactions sound too difficult to you at first, start by taking baby steps. Join a support group for people who are dealing with the same struggles as you. Overeaters Anonymous (which is what Mary Jo Schneider, profiled in chapter 1, relied on) is a good example. Or you could try an online support system such as the message boards on www.thebestlife.com. These are great because they allow you to interact and socialize in a more comfortable, nonintimidating way. Many of the Best Life members have developed strong friendships online and have even gone on to meet up in person to bond and share their experiences and lessons.

BARRIER: A LIMITED VISION OF YOURSELF

After years of being put down—by others and yourself—you simply come to accept these criticisms as truth: You're too fat to do anything. You'll never lose weight. No one will ever love you as long as you look like that. Whether these words came from a parent while you were growing up, a spouse, or even yourself, the result is the same: You feel boxed in or controlled by an outdated or distorted image of yourself. The truth is, no one ever changes or improves if she accepts these beliefs. Obtaining a healthy body image requires letting yourself feel vulnerable. But the payoff is huge—a major life transformation can take place.

Take a few minutes once a month to read the questions below and jot down your answers in a notebook or journal. You can use the sample exercise below as a guide before you fill out your own answers in the spaces provided.

SAMPLE

1. *What is your current shell (the job, the habits, the expectations that bind you)?*
Example: I'm a jolly fat guy who always has a joke to share and will make everyone laugh. I'm also the good guy who never says no and whom everyone likes.

2. *Do you need to discard your shell?*
Example: Yes.

3. *Are you afraid to discard your shell? If so, why?*
Example: Yes. I'm worried that people will see that I'm not so jolly, that they won't like me when I say no and decide to do more for myself, and that my wife will feel vulnerable and threatened if I lose weight. And I'm afraid that if I lose weight, I'll end up having affairs like my dad did.

4. *What would you lose if you discarded your shell?*
Example: The safety of being the "jolly fat guy."

THE LOBSTER LESSON

Marianne Larson had been a schoolteacher who took early retirement at age sixty so she could help take care of her grandchildren. But she realized early into her retirement that after twenty years of teaching young children, she didn't want to spend four days a week babysitting. She wanted to do things she never had time to do when she was working full-time and raising a family, like take classes, paint, and form a book club.

However, she felt selfish for experiencing these feelings, because she knew her daughter was counting on her, and she didn't want to disappoint her. So Marianne watched her grandchildren, binged on the snacks she fed them, and began to feel depressed as she gained 25 pounds. She sought treatment because she had become increasingly depressed and withdrawn from others.

In our therapy, Marianne shared that she had suffered severe physical abuse at the hands of her father, and because of this, she had become adept at reading what he and others needed and meeting those needs. As a child, she'd learned that if she was "good" and did what her father expected, she could avoid provoking him. As Marianne grew up, her need to pacify and please went beyond her father—she didn't want to disappoint *anyone* and would do almost anything to keep people from getting angry with her.

It was not surprising to me when she realized that she was afraid to tell her daughter that she didn't want to spend her retirement as the primary babysitter for her grandkids. She did what victims of childhood abuse often do: She didn't see a way out, so she found a way to get through it. Common compensatory behaviors include drinking or spending too much money, engaging in risky behaviors, and—in Marianne's case—overeating and bingeing.

Our therapy focused on helping Marianne understand the effects of abuse and developing the capacity to be assertive and speak up for herself. Marianne realized that when she told her daughter that she wanted to watch the kids only one day a week, her daughter might be disappointed, even angry. She didn't feel ready to talk to her daughter just yet, so I urged her to continue to work on putting herself and her needs first and accepting this possible outcome.

One evening, Marianne and her husband went out to dinner with their daughter and her family. They were waiting in line next to a tank with lobsters. Her son-in-law had minored in oceanography in college and loved to talk about sea creatures. He began to tell her all about the lobsters in the tank. "Lobsters must molt in order to grow. As the lobster gets larger, it needs to grow a more spacious shell," he explained. "This soft creature that is used to having a strong armor around it now must go out into the world exposed. They might be eaten by prey or washed up on the reef and die. The period between shells is one where the lobster is vulnerable but must go through in order to grow."

After this conversation, Marianne dreamt about lobsters every night. There would be lobsters on her table, lobsters walking in line after her, lobsters staring at her. She said, "Not only am I depressed and overeating, but I am crazy, too." With some help, Marianne realized that the lobster was a metaphor for herself. She'd outgrown her shell. But she was afraid to discard the shell and let others know what she really wanted to do.

Shortly after that dinner, Marianne met with her daughter to tell her she'd only be able to watch the kids one day a week so she could pursue her other interests. Her daughter was disappointed and angry at first. She told Marianne that no one could take care of the grandkids like their grandmother. Marianne listened to her daughter's concerns and feelings, but she was assertive and explained that this was something she needed to do for herself.

In our next session, Marianne and I talked about the fact that if we lived in an ideal world, those who are closest to you would be supportive of you when you make choices to take care of your body and yourself. But we live in the real world, where people are sometimes angry because they're used to you always saying yes and putting their needs before your own. I explained to her that although it may be difficult to put yourself first, you have to do it. Marianne found that after her daughter's initial anger subsided, they were able to work together to find a good babysitter for the kids through their church. Marianne felt better about her relationship with her daughter after they got through this conflict. She realized that she no longer had to be that scared child who had to please everyone or risk abuse. Her eating improved, and she became more active, walking with other retired teachers five days a week. Marianne learned that to really grow and learn, you have to allow yourself to be vulnerable, to lose your shell.

5. *What would you gain if you discarded your shell?*
Example: I would gain respect for myself, respect from others, and—without my armor of fat—maybe grow closer to my wife and be taken more seriously by others.

Now it's your turn:

1. *What is your current shell (the job, the habits, the expectations that bind you)?*

_____

2. *Do you need to discard your shell?*

_____

3. *Are you afraid to discard your shell? If so, why?*

_____

4. *What would you lose if you discarded your shell?*

_____

5. *What would you gain if you discarded your shell?*

_____

In order to develop a different relationship with your body, you need to leave behind excess baggage and/or outdated versions of yourself. You must be courageous and take a big leap to let go of the old and make way for the new—to finally see your body as an important source of information (about hunger, satiety, when you need to rest or slow down) and of pleasure and love.

Just as it's important to periodically clean your closet of clothes that no longer fit, you must also get rid of negative thoughts and images of your body that leave you depressed and unmotivated. Change can be downright uncomfortable at times, but don't forget how painful it is to be locked into a negative body image, how it limits your motivation, your confidence in relationships with others, and possibly your career. You may be holding yourself back at work or you may be missing out on the opportunity to let others love you and become close to you because you are forever judging and being critical of your body.

It's time for you to shed your shell and be free of a negative body image. You may be scared or feel unprotected, but you won't be vulnerable forever. Eventually you'll grow a new shell, and the new way that you relate to food, your body, and others will start to feel like home. Remember, not changing is often harder than changing. Consider your options: Stay stuck and stagnant with a negative body image for the rest of your life or do some tough emotional work so you can accept, understand, and love yourself for who you are and finally achieve all your weight, health, and life goals.

Your body image is a crucial element of how you feel about yourself. Though it can be related to your weight, simply dropping pounds won't improve your body image—you must first learn how to love and appreciate your body regardless of its appearance. Addressing the barriers described throughout this chapter and completing the sample exercises will help you to develop a new perspective on your body. If you've unsuccessfully attempted weight loss before, it's time to set a new, attainable weight loss goal. Be realistic about your goal weight, make time for yourself to meet it, and follow through with your plan to the best of your ability.

While you're on the path toward a healthier lifestyle, it's important to remind yourself that appearance isn't *everything*. Weight-related prejudice is real and can be hurtful, but do not let your weight dictate what you do and where you go in life. Start working on improving your body image today. It will facilitate your weight loss efforts and allow you to feel deserving of a happy, fulfilled life.

6

MAINTAINING WEIGHT LOSS: WHAT WORKS AND WHAT DOESN'T

By Bob Greene

IF THERE IS ONE thing that's true for almost everyone who has ever lost a significant number of pounds, it's that the work doesn't stop there. You have to *keep* eating carefully and *keep* being physically active. You have to keep on top of your attitudes and emotional health, too.

The previous chapters were aimed at both motivating you to tackle the barriers standing in the way of weight loss and giving you direction on how to do it. But as you go forward, it's also important to know how to keep the weight you lose from coming back. Part of that, I believe, will be inherent in the approach to weight loss that we have just laid out for you. When you knock down the emotional and psychological barriers (and learn to cope with the physiological ones) that prevented you from being successful in the first place, you're going to have a much greater shot at keeping the pounds from returning.

Still, there are practical matters that make a difference, too, and for that it's instructive to look at how successful maintainers manage to prevent weight regain. So let's examine the National Weight Control Registry, the large, ongoing research study that I mentioned in the beginning of this book. To refresh your memory, membership in this "club" is predicated on having lost at least thirty pounds and having kept it off for at least a year. (Some of its members, you may have noticed, have been profiled throughout this book.) Many of the participants, who range in age from eighteen to ninety-one and come from all walks of life, have actually lost a lot more than that and maintained it far longer. It's impressive, but don't chalk them up as the lucky few. Ninety percent of them tried to lose weight and failed many times before eventually triumphing over excess pounds.

When you listen to what successful maintainers say about their ultimate success, it's clear that for many of them, weight loss went hand in hand with making monumental changes in their lives. Some got out of bad relationships, some switched careers, some learned how to set boundaries with others—whatever the change was, it was often significant. And what drove them to change varied from person to person. For about a third of the NWCR participants, the "lightbulb" moment was health related: Sleep apnea (when you stop breathing for short periods during sleep), an aching back, heart disease, diabetes, or another weight-related condition propelled their desire to do what it took to finally lose weight. Another third took an emotional hit before they got really serious about weight loss; discovering that their spouses left them because of their weight jolted them into action. Some were motivated by special events such as weddings and class reunions, or by seeing themselves in a full-length mirror, or not being able to fit in their clothes any longer. The point is, there was no one universal "aha" moment. Just as we've encouraged you to do throughout this book, all of them found an incentive that spoke to them personally, then they followed through.

So what else helped them succeed and, more specifically (and importantly), stay the course? Here are seven strategies that worked for successful maintainers—and will work for you, too.

THEY REALLY MOVE

You don't have to participate in a triathlon, break the record at your gym for the number of consecutive pull-ups, or win the police academy Physical Training Award like Shaun Tympanick (see box, page 21) to keep your weight off, but you do have to be active—very active. On average, NWCR participants burn 2,621 calories weekly from going to the gym, jogging, or other types of sporting or recreational activity, as well as from walking and taking the stairs as much as possible.

Maintainers actually exercise longer and harder than people who've never been overweight. In one study, they worked out an average of about sixty minutes daily compared to fifty-two minutes for the never-overweight group. The difference in workout intensity was even more telling: Maintainers averaged twenty-four minutes daily of moderately high-intensity activity compared to about seventeen minutes for the never overweight. Over weeks and months, that adds up to a big difference in calories burned. While not every successful maintainer strength trains, the NWCR data show that the numbers of those who do are growing. I'm not surprised. Strength training increases the rate at which you burn calories. Cardio exercise is great, and it's where many people who want to lose weight start, but if you really want to have the ultimate workout plan, you'll need to incorporate strength training as well. Follow my exercise guidelines in chapter 4, and you'll be on track to duplicate the maintainers' success, then check out appendix 6 for a sample plan that consists of both strength and cardio. *The lesson here is that if you want to lose weight and keep it off, you're going to have to step up your activity—there's no way around it.*

THEY'RE HEALTHY EATERS

You probably were expecting this one. Yes, successful maintainers do eat nutritiously and in moderation. Here are some specifics:

- *They keep a lid on calories.* The average reported calorie count of NWCR participants is 1,380 per day—although that number warrants a little explanation. "Our participants report their calorie intake, we don't measure it directly, and studies consistently show that people tend to underestimate their calorie intake by about 30 percent," says Suzanne Phelan, PhD, a psychologist who is one of the principal NWCR researchers as well as an assistant professor of kinesiology at California Polytechnic State University. Underestimating by 30 percent would make the actual daily count a much more satisfying and doable 1,800 calories. And it's an average; some people need more calories, others less. Whatever you determine is right for you; the point is that you can't go back to your old high-calorie ways.

- *They're careful.* Successful maintainers score high in what nutritionists and psychologists call "dietary restraint": behaviors such as doling out small portions of food, avoiding high-calorie foods, and counting calories or grams of fat. "The first thing I do when I pick up a food," says Shaun Tympanick, "is look at the nutrition label and check out the calories. That doesn't mean I'll eat only low-calorie foods—I'll still have chips or chocolate on occasion—but I know just how much I can eat."

- *They eat a balanced diet.* For the most part, the successful maintainers' diets follow the recommendations of the American Heart Association and other major health organizations. About 54 percent of calories come from carbohydrates (including five to six servings of fruits and vegetables daily), about 27 percent from fat, and about 19 percent from protein.

- *They eat breakfast.* Nearly 100 percent of NWCR participants eat breakfast, with most of them doing so every day of the week. That's in sharp contrast to the 25 percent of Americans who are breakfast skippers. Need some quick and easy breakfast ideas? Check out my website, www.thebestlife.com—the recipe database is loaded with hundreds of delicious and fresh meal ideas.

- *They steer clear of drive-thrus.* Fast food may have helped them pack on the pounds, but once they lost the weight, successful maintainers largely avoid it, eating, on average, less than one fast-food meal a week. "My sister and I used to go out for fast food and buffets all the time, but we just don't do that anymore," says Terane Weatherly, whose story is featured on page 146.

THEY LIMIT THEIR DIETARY OPTIONS

Talk to a nutritionist, and sooner or later she'll say the word *variety,* as in: Eat a variety of fruits and vegetables to get the most nutrients; eat various types of whole grains to get different types of fiber; vary your meals so you don't get bored. But if you want to take a page from people who keep weight off, maybe your diet shouldn't be *too* exciting. Dr. Phelan and her co-researchers compared the diets of NWCR members with those of people who recently lost weight but had no track record of maintaining. These newly minted "losers" were a good comparison group because they had to clean up their diets to lose the weight, eating more fruits and vegetables and less junky high-fat food. The striking difference between maintainers and those who'd recently slimmed down: The maintainers ate less variety. And they didn't just limit their picks of sweets (as well as oils, butter, and other fats); they also had a slightly downsized repertoire of foods in the vegetable, low-fat protein, and grain groups.

These findings aren't that surprising. By limiting variety, you can more easily control your body's natural inclination to seek different tastes and flavors. As Janis explained in detail in chapter 3, this is a trait that kept our ancestors alive, ensuring that they ate a variety of foods, which helped them get a variety of nutrients. Just think of how much more you put on your plate at a buffet than when you order a la carte. Or how there always seems to be room for dessert, no matter how full you are.

Shaun Tympanick keeps a lid on variety. "My fridge is really plain Jane," he says, "with just the basics: skim milk, low-fat cheese, seltzer, egg whites in a carton, and Lean Cuisine frozen meals. I'll try new things, but I don't like to have too much around to tempt me." The takeaway here is that while you don't want a diet so boring that you go back to your old habits, you also don't want one that's so varied it triggers overeating. *Sticking with a consistent group of healthy foods and a regular eating schedule (no cheat days) will help you keep the weight off.*

THEY TURN OFF THE TUBE

Thirty-five hours: That's the amount of time the average American spends per week watching TV. After work and sleep, TV viewing takes up more time than any other activity in the United States. But not for NWCR participants. Sixty-two percent watch less than ten hours weekly, and a third watch less than five hours. While the average American is sitting in front of the TV (and, often, snacking), successful weight maintainers might be taking an after-dinner walk, whipping up a healthy meal, or working out at the gym. And even if they're just walking around the house doing chores, they're still burning a lot more calories than they would if they were sitting in front of the television. They're also subject to less temptation. A 2009 Yale University study found that adults consumed an extra 150 calories of snacks after watching TV shows that contained food ads compared to programs that ran none.

The message is clear: *The less time you spend in front of a screen (TV, computer, or video-game), the higher your odds of maintaining your weight loss.*

WHAT DOESN'T WORK

While most participants in the National Weight Control Registry maintained their weight loss after initially registering with the study, 35 percent of them actually relapsed, regaining an average of fifteen and a half pounds (although some regained only about five pounds). What went wrong? Fortunately, researchers were there to document which factors contributed to the weight gain. You can learn a lot from the maintainers' mistakes as well as note that some issues leading to relapse (such as emotional eating and depression) may warrant seeking professional help. Here's what the NWCR researchers discovered:

Relapsers
— ate inconsistently, with low-calorie and higher-calorie swings;
— hit fast-food joints more often;
— watched more TV;
— skipped breakfast;
— were more likely to suffer from emotional eating;
— were more prone to depression.

THEY KEEP CLOSE WATCH ON THEIR WEIGHT, NIPPING ANY GAIN IN THE BUD

The bathroom scales of successful maintainers aren't collecting dust: They weigh themselves at least once a week. What seems to work best for maintenance is establishing a regular weigh-in routine that works for you—whether it's daily, weekly, or a little less often—and sticking with it. What didn't work for NWCR participants: going from frequent weigh-ins to less frequent checks. Over a year's time, those who stopped weighing themselves as often as they used to gained nine pounds, compared to four pounds for people who didn't change their weighing routine. But it's not only a decrease in the frequency of weigh-ins that's a problem: Any adjustment seemed to be accompanied by weight gain. For instance, those who decided to step on the scale even *more* frequently than they usually did gained slightly over two pounds.

Regular weigh-ins are a good idea when you're in the maintenance phase, but I caution clients about using the scale during the initial stages of weight loss. During this time, the body is adjusting to eating healthier and exercising more, and the numbers on the scale often don't reflect these changes. Not only does your weight naturally fluctuate in the first few weeks after starting a weight loss plan, but I find that people are most vulnerable during this period. The scale can wreak havoc in the initial stages of weight loss: You're working hard and making tough changes, and if you don't see results right away, that can be very frustrating.

My recommendation: *Weigh yourself when you first begin a weight loss program for a baseline, or starting point. Then hold off for four weeks before stepping on the scale again.* After that, you should keep tabs on your weight on a more regular basis. I recommend once a week. (To get the most accurate reading, try to weigh yourself on the same day each week, at the same time, using the same scale and wearing the same clothes.) In fact, the scale is a reliable early warning signal that something's amiss with either your diet or exercise habits. When the numbers go up, you have an opportunity to fine-tune your diet or exercise regimen. If you know that the numbers on the scale tend to make you nutty, try using a pair of pants as a gauge instead. If they get too tight, maybe it's time to tighten the reins on your diet and/or fitness plan.

THEY DON'T EAT FOR EMOTIONAL REASONS

Given the prevalence of emotional eating in the general population, it's safe to assume that a large portion of maintainers struggled with emotional eating. Indeed, most of the people profiled in this book who've kept off the weight they lost admit to dealing with emotional eating. To examine just how big a problem it is, Brown University researchers gave NWCR members a questionnaire assessing the degree and type of emotional eating they were prone to, then checked in on them a year later. They did the same for a group of men and women who'd recently lost weight on a diet and exercise program called TRIM. (This group didn't have a maintenance track record yet.) In both groups, those who had the biggest emotional eating problems gained back the most weight. Still, NWCR participants scored lower—in other words, had less severe emotional eating and gained back less weight—than those enrolled in TRIM, which is probably why they were able to make it into the NWCR in the first place.

The statistics are clear: *If you want to get your weight under control, you're going to have to eliminate emotional eating, just as Ann helps you do in chapter 2.*

SURGICAL OPTIONS: WHEN YOUR BEST EFFORTS DON'T WORK

For some people, cutting calories and increasing activity as well as doing the emotional work required to remedy the issues that led to weight gain in the first place aren't enough. They just can't lose weight. In many of these cases, bariatric surgery may be an option.

Bariatric surgery is a blanket term for many different procedures, including gastric bypass and lap-band surgery. I'm not recommending any of the procedures for everyone, or even for anyone who can't seem to overcome nature's will. But if your body weight poses significant danger to your health—that is, if the risks of staying obese outweigh the risks of surgery and the lingering side effects—then you may want to consider surgery.

The procedures have been shown to be quite literally lifesavers for certain people. In one study, people who had a BMI of at least 35 (which is considered obese) and underwent weight loss surgery were 40 percent less likely than obese people who didn't have the surgery to die from any cause—including heart disease, cancer, and diabetes—seven years after the procedure.

Bariatric surgery has gotten some bad press, probably because too many people who could trim down with diet and exercise are opting for the surgical solution. But on the flip side, many people who would probably benefit most from the surgery aren't getting it.

In fact, of the fifteen million Americans with a BMI over 40 (which is considered morbidly obese), only 1 percent undergoes bariatric surgery. Of course, no surgery is without risks or complications, and that's true for this type of surgery as well. In addition to the risks *during* surgery, there are also lasting side effects after the procedure, such as an inability to absorb certain vitamins and minerals and an intolerance to specific foods.

Finally, the surgeries are not a guarantee against future weight gain. Research from McGill University in Canada suggests that 20 percent to 35 percent of gastric bypass surgeries are considered failures because of weight regain after ten years. In a separate study published in the medical journal *Obesity Surgery*, 79 percent of patients who had undergone bariatric surgery reported weight regain—though only a third of them regained a significant amount. ("Significant" was defined as 15 percent of the weight they'd lost. For instance, if someone lost one hundred pounds and gained back fifteen or more pounds, it was considered significant.) Further research from Switzerland indicates that 40 percent to 45 percent of people fail to achieve sufficient weight loss two years after having the lap-band surgery partly because of complications.

Are you a candidate? The National Institutes of Health recommends meeting these three criteria:

1. A body mass index (BMI) of 40 or more, which represents about one hundred pounds overweight for men and eighty pounds for women. A lower BMI, between 35 and 39.9, is also considered an appropriate criterion if it's accompanied by a serious obesity-related health problem such as type 2 diabetes, coronary heart disease, or severe sleep apnea. To find out your BMI, turn to appendix 2.

2. You are healthy enough to withstand the operation without a high likelihood of major complications.

3. After the surgery, you also must be able and willing to exercise and to cut back on eating. Counseling is highly recommended; otherwise the weight will likely come back.

The two most common types of bariatric surgery are the adjustable gastric band (AGB), or lap band, and gastric bypass (also called Roux-en-Y gastric bypass, or RYGB). The point of AGB surgery is to shrink the normally football-sized stomach to the size of a golf ball by wrapping a silicone band around it, making it impossible to eat very much at any one sitting. However, with time, you can stretch the stomach, and if you're not careful, you can override the band, regaining weight.

The second procedure, gastric bypass, involves connecting the stomach to the middle of the small intestine. (It normally attaches to the first of the three sections of the small intestine.) Food is typically broken down and absorbed at the beginning of the small bowel, so if you bypass a large portion of it, you reduce the number of calorie-containing nutrients (carbs, protein, fat, and alcohol) that the body can absorb. In addition, the stomach is sewn, leaving just a small pouch. As with lap-band surgery, the stomach can stretch, so it's possible to undo the effects of this operation by overeating. However, because the procedure also helps limit calorie absorption, it's more effective than AGB. That's why gastric bypass makes up 80 percent of all bariatric surgeries. There is an even more drastic version of this operation, in which the stomach is connected even farther down the small intestine, so you absorb very little of your meals. That procedure, called biliopancreatic diversion with duodenal switch, is riskier and rarely performed.

THEY DON'T HAVE A PERFECTIONIST MENTALITY

Judging yourself to be either "on" or "off" a diet, or "bad" or "good," is a typical pitfall for people trying to maintain weight loss. On the other hand, cutting yourself some slack and getting right back on track when you veer off the path is a common attitude among successful maintainers—and not only those among the NWCR group. Researchers at the University of Western Australia, for instance, found that 73 percent of people who gained back lost weight were black-and-white perfectionist thinkers, as compared to just 7 percent of weight maintainers.

It's so easy to gain back the weight when every little cookie or missed workout signals failure. The occasional rich dessert, the business trip that interferes with your gym day, or other ways you stumble are normal and inevitable. To survive them, you'll have to roll with it. Says Jennifer Demuth, profiled on page 150, "I allow myself regular little indulgences like ice cream, birthday cake, chocolate, and French fries. The key is that my indulgences are only in small portions and aren't an everyday thing."

Strangely enough, I've found that some people who are prone to perfectionist thinking are actually subconsciously waiting for a slipup (a twisted ankle, a bad eating day) so they have a reason or excuse for returning to their bad habits. If you subscribe to the all-or-nothing train of thought, you'll need to give yourself an attitude adjustment. *Slipups are inevitable. You'll need to be somewhat flexible and forgiving if you're going to stay the course.*

GOOD NEWS! IT GETS EASIER

If losing weight is or has been a struggle, and your attempts at maintenance have been no picnic, here's some welcome news: The longer you maintain, the easier it gets. Former drug or alcohol abusers have the same experience. The longer they stay clean, the less likely they are to relapse. Two years seemed to be the magic number for NWCR participants. If they stuck it out for that long, their odds of gaining back five or more pounds were cut in half. Those who maintained for five years had even better odds: just a 30 percent chance of gaining back more than five pounds.

As they say, old habits die hard—but they *do* die if you work at it, and I think that successful losers prove that point. After a certain amount of time, preparing a healthy meal at home, ordering the leaner dish at a restaurant, or making it to the gym doesn't feel like a big deal anymore. "The longer people eat well and exercise, the more these may become ingrained habits that require less conscious effort," explains Dr. Phelan.

There is also some other positive news about maintaining weight loss. Ninety-five percent of the NWCR successful losers say that their quality of life has improved. They have more energy, an improved mood, and increased self-confidence. Most of them also reported that their relationships with spouses, friends, the opposite sex, parents, and strangers also improved.

If you go back and read the stories of Terane Weatherly, Mary Jo Schneider, and Shaun Tympanick, it's obvious that losing weight dramatically bettered their lives in ways they appreciate. But it's also important to note that I've seen plenty of people lose weight—sometimes well over one hundred pounds—yet *not* really appreciate it. They're lighter, they move better, they're more socially active, but when really pushed, they can't see or enjoy how much their life has improved because they're still hung up on the issue that caused their weight gain in the first place. So the weight, which is often a symptom of a bigger problem, might go away, but the problem (a bad relationship, an inability to set boundaries, pain you suffered as a child, feeling unworthy of happiness) remains until it's addressed. I can't stress how crucial this is: *People who slim down the right way are happier overall, and they appreciate the fact that their life is better. That makes staying motivated to maintain these changes so much easier.*

MEASURING SUCCESS

In this chapter, I've used the word *successful* a lot. But what exactly is success? For the National Weight Control Registry, it's the criteria I described earlier: losing at least thirty pounds and maintaining that loss for at least a year. For your doctor, it might be maintaining a loss of 5 percent or 10 percent of your body weight, just enough to lower blood pressure or blood sugar or improve your health in some other way. I tend to view success in terms of improved health *and* happiness—that is, you live life in a way that not only puts you at a healthier weight but also brings more joy into your life. Happiness is such an important piece of the puzzle, as Ann will make clear in the following chapter.

How *you* define weight loss success is critical to your, well, success going forward. To feel like you're a successful maintainer, you must first be more or less comfortable with the weight you're maintaining. And you don't even have to get all the way down to your goal weight to be satisfied. You can still be happy and comfortable with weight loss even if you fall short of this mark. To do that, you have to understand and accept your body and your genetics. Once you accept your shape, life gets a whole lot easier. Then you can maintain a weight that's healthy but realistic, without having to make sacrifices that would detract from your overall happiness. As Ann explains, "This weight might not be the number you initially had in mind, but it's the point at which you're comfortable with your weight and shape and are still able to do all the things that are important to you, such as travel, play with your kids, hike, and so on.

"Having a healthy life requires balance," she continues, "and you can't have balance when losing more weight would require having to eat so little or exercise so much that you would not be able to engage in other important aspects of your life."

In fact, many people eventually settle in at a slightly higher (but just as healthy) weight than they'd originally planned. Consider that you will probably never be rail thin (and this is the case for about 98 percent of Americans, by the way), and that it's okay. Your genes might dictate that you will be solid and muscular or curvy. When you set your goal weight, remember to consider all the factors that affect weight, including genetics, your body shape and muscle mass, and how you functioned at various weight levels. For instance, if you struggled to maintain 140 pounds in the past, but were just as healthy— and much happier—at 150, then you may have to adjust your goal weight up slightly.

No matter what you weigh now or what weight you're trying to get to, it's crucial that you look beyond the scale for measures of success. There is, for instance, that improved lab report from your doctor and the sense of satisfaction you get from looking better in your clothes, or simply feeling better. Exercise milestones are especially satisfying—progress from five-pound weights to fifteen-pound weights, and you've tripled your strength! And how gratifying is it to double your miles on the treadmill? Being able to walk your dog, play with your children, have the energy to cook a healthful meal when you get home from work, do anything that you once couldn't—there are so many ways to mark achievement. Continue to strive for the things you want and deserve in life and congratulate yourself for every barrier you knock down and every triumph (big and small) along the way. Many, myself included, believe that the ultimate success is being happy, as it is a reflection of all that is important and meaningful to you in this life.

7

BEING HAPPY

By Ann Kearney-Cooke

TO BE SUCCESSFUL AT losing weight and maintaining that loss, you have to do more than simply count calories and stick to a regular workout schedule—this is a key theme that we keep coming back to throughout this book. Overcoming barriers, such as our physiological wiring, emotional eating, and poor body image, are also vital to the process of slimming down and staying that way. But there's one more important factor that you can't overlook: finding pleasure, happiness, and fulfillment in your day-to-day life.

Being happy might seem like a bonus or side effect of losing weight—the end result of all your hard work. Many people mistakenly believe that they'll be happier once they've shed pounds. But being happy—or, more specifically, finding sources of happiness in your life on a daily basis—is more like a prerequisite for taking off the weight. In fact, you could even say that the essence of motivation is in finding happiness in moving toward your goals, or in the pursuit of happiness. For instance, taking even small steps, such as going for a ten-minute walk or packing a healthy snack so that you don't raid the vending machine at work, can be very satisfying. But many people simply aren't able to find joy in these types of accomplishments because they're too busy obsessing about something else: often the fact that they're not burning enough calories or losing weight quickly enough. Sure, that short walk or healthy snack choice is probably just a drop in the bucket, but the act itself reinforces the belief that you're worth it, that you deserve to be nurtured. These little acts, which can bring small hits of happiness, are the fuel for motivation.

Unfortunately, sometimes the weight loss process itself can be detrimental to long-term weight loss success and, ultimately, your happiness, particularly if you *do* focus too much on losing weight and ignore other important areas of your life. Bob has often said that people mistakenly put all their emotional eggs in the weight-loss basket, so inevitably, when weight loss slows or stops, they fail to get the emotional high that they used to get from seeing the numbers on the scale drop. They may then look to other areas of their life for this sense of satisfaction, but because they've ignored these areas, they're left frustrated. As a result, they often return to their old habits.

Happiness involves recognizing all the areas of your life that are important to you—not just your eating or fitness routine—and actively working on improving them to the best of your ability each day. If it helps, you can write down all the factors that are essential to a happy, fulfilled life, and then mark down those that are doing well and those that may be falling short of your expectations, so you know what you need to work on. The simple act of paying attention to your needs and nurturing yourself (and others) is a powerful source of joy, fulfillment, and happiness. And when you're able to derive a sense of pleasure from caring for yourself and taking small steps toward improving your life, you'll find that good health and happiness come more easily.

Another mistake people can make when it comes to happiness is thinking of it as a black-or-white issue. It's not like you're going to reach a point in your life where suddenly you think, *Wow, I'm happy!* Rather, as you work toward achieving goals in life—whether they're losing weight, exercising, eating healthfully, or developing positive relationships with others—you have to be able to take pleasure from the process. If you don't find sources of pleasure and joy along the way, one of two things typically happen. Either you'll lose the motivation to continue on your healthier path or you'll achieve your goals but struggle to maintain them.

And of course, when you're feeling happy, satisfied, and fulfilled as you work toward any type of goal, you'll have more energy and motivation, which makes continuing to make these lifestyle changes easier. On the other hand, nothing can drain your energy and kill motivation like feeling down or blue, being in a persistent funk, or experiencing clinical depression. Prolonged feelings of sadness, depression, and/or lethargy can also lead to a relapse in people who have successfully maintained significant weight loss for years. That's why in this chapter, I'll be sharing information taken from research studies and from my experience working with clients on how to live a happy, more satisfying life.

THE HISTORY OF HAPPINESS

Happiness is not some elusive feeling or unattainable goal. Thanks to real, scientific data, we now know what makes people happy in general, and how you can use your talents and strengths to achieve happiness in your own life. The field of positive psychology was born in the late 1990s, when psychologist Martin Seligman encouraged his colleagues to begin researching mental wellness with the same scientific vigor they'd long used to study mental illness. The focus was to learn how to make life more fulfilling and increase well-being. At the same time, the field of neurobiology emerged and provided more clues as to what makes people happy. Research using MRI and PET (positron-emission topography) scans has taught us a great deal about the brain states that underlie positive moods and how we can influence the brain through mental interventions.

It didn't take long for the interest in happiness to make the jump from the lab to the general public. In 2000 only fifty books on the topic of happiness were published; in 2008 the number jumped to four thousand. Positive psychology workshops began popping up across the country. Currently, one of the most popular classes at many universities focuses on findings from positive psychologists about how to live a happy life. Even the Dalai Lama has written about the importance of happiness; two of his books on the subject were released in the 1990s; the third one came out in 2009. The main argument of these books is that the purpose of life is to be happy. He asserts that happiness is not a hobby or trivial pursuit, it is a basic, fundamental human drive.

It might seem odd to lump happiness in there with other basic needs, such as food and water. After all, happiness is somewhat vague and subjective; what makes one person happy might not necessarily work for another. But there are some criteria when it comes to determining what makes people happy and why. In my work, I've come to understand happiness as the point at which you can handle the ups and downs of life without becoming too attached to the good or victimized by the bad—when you can keep an open heart, be compassionate toward others, live in the moment, and be fully present as you carry out your day-to-day activities. You are happiest when you feel that your life is purposeful and that it makes a difference—be it in the life of your child or in the world at large. Finally, creating a life that is full of activities that are surprising, dynamic, and fun contributes significantly to happiness.

THE SCIENCE OF HAPPINESS

Studies looking into happiness have uncovered a number of interesting findings, including:

- Whether you win the lottery or become paralyzed by a spinal cord injury, you will tend to be, on average, no more or less happy a year later. Despite the occurrence of positive or negative life events, people generally return to their baseline levels of happiness relatively quickly.

- Can money buy happiness? Research shows that having enough money is crucial to happiness. Financial stress can stand in the way of enjoying life; having enough money to alleviate this stress can go a long way toward increasing your happiness. However, more isn't necessarily better. After your basic needs are met (food, shelter, safety) and you have a little left over as a cushion, extra material wealth has little to no effect on life satisfaction or happiness.

- Age seems to bring not only wisdom but happiness, too. Older people are more satisfied with their lives than younger people. A recent survey by the Centers for Disease Control and Prevention found that people in their early twenties are sad for an average of 3.4 days per month as opposed to just 2.3 days per month for people ages sixty-five to seventy-four. Freed from child rearing and the stress of building and maintaining a career, older adults have more time to pursue their own interests. Not to mention, as you age, you gain wisdom, perspective, and emotional intelligence, all of which can help you deal with life's challenges and stresses more efficiently.

- Want to be happier? Say "I do." People in steady relationships are generally happier than those who are single. Healthy romantic relationships provide elements that contribute to happiness, such as companionship, support, security, intimacy, and self-growth.

HAPPINESS HOW-TO

What makes one person happier than another? Believe it or not, it may have as much or more to do with genetics than your current life status. There are three primary factors that determine how happy a person is, according to happiness researcher Sonja Lyubomirsky, PhD. Her research indicates that 50 percent of individual differences are genetic. Studies of identical twins suggest the blueprint for happiness is in our genes, so if you come from a family that tends to be more happy and cheerful, you probably will be, too. How we think and what we do—our actions and behaviors as well as our outlook—account for 40 percent of individual differences. And only 10 percent can be attributed to a person's life circumstances, such as where you live or what your job is.

A study from the *Journal of Happiness Studies* supports her research: The study's authors asked people to report various acts of recent positive changes in their activities (such as starting a new fitness program) versus positive changes in their circumstances (such as moving to a nicer house). The researchers discovered that activity-based changes accurately predicted well-being both six and twelve weeks after the start of the study. Circumstance-based change predicted well-being only at six weeks. It appears that by the twelfth week, individuals had already adapted to their circumstantial changes, while the benefits of their activity-based changes continued to contribute to greater contentment. The take-home message: What matters more in terms of happiness are the small decisions you make each day. The bigger things—your life circumstances, which are often harder to change—have a fleeting and less significant effect.

That also means that even if you got shortchanged in the genetic lottery, there's still a lot you can do to live a happier life. In fact, a full 40 percent of your capacity for happiness is completely in your hands. It's those everyday decisions you make that can infuse your life with more happiness and joy. So what kind of choices do you need to make to increase feelings of satisfaction and well-being in your life? Use the plan below to live a happier, more purposeful life.

YOUR PLAN FOR INCREASING HAPPINESS

Maintain Healthy Relationships

Connecting with others by engaging in healthy relationships is one of the most important sources of happiness. Relationships strengthen the belief that you're not alone, no matter how difficult your life is. The ability to work with and lean on others during tough times and to celebrate important, positive life transitions is crucial for living with vitality and joy.

Most of us have been seduced by the American dream that anyone can get rich and that riches reap happiness. However, obtaining material possessions often requires working long hours, which translates into lost time with family and friends. Initially, the material rewards can be exciting and gratifying—but these feelings deteriorate over time. Think about the first time you got a new car or bought a house. It was an exhilarating and joyful experience. But as time passed, the adrenaline wore off, and you returned to your normal state. In fact, you might have ended up feeling worse: depleted and stressed because paying off this purchase likely lasted much longer than the happiness associated with buying it. Remember, very few material possessions improve with age. A new house does not stay new for long before trips to Home Depot and calls to repairmen become more frequent. And a car starts to lose its value the second you drive it off the lot.

On the other hand, researchers have found that satisfaction with interpersonal experiences tends to increase over time; relationships with people simply have more enduring value. A family reunion with relatives of all ages enjoying meals together, sharing rich stories of the past and present, and celebrating the family's new additions can live on as a source of joy for years to come—much longer than that pricey car or costly home.

So take a look at your social connections with friends, family, coworkers, neighbors, and groups. Some of these relationships may not qualify as healthy and therefore will not be consistent sources of happiness and fulfillment—in fact, they can significantly detract from your happiness and fulfillment. Healthy relationships are based on trust, honesty, equality, good communication, and separate identities. You feel as comfortable doing things to nurture and care for yourself as you would doing these things for your partner. You feel accepted for who you are and have the freedom to be close to others outside the relationship. You are close but separate, have your privacy, and can say no without fear of abandonment or hostility.

Of course, there's no such thing as a perfect relationship. We all enter relationships with our own emotional baggage and unfinished business from the past. Feelings of disappointment, fear, and sadness can be part of any relationship at some point. But when your relationship is more about discomfort, fear, and pain than about mutual respect and growth, you need to take action. If you feel a particular relationship is causing you more pain than joy, it's important to voice your concerns and be specific about what your friend or partner is doing that's making you unhappy. You must be clear about what has to change and what you're willing to negotiate to be more satisfied in the relationship. In some cases, you may need a professional, such as a therapist, to help you make the necessary changes to get your relationship back on track.

If the other person is not willing to work on improving the relationship, you may need to consider ending it. You shouldn't stay in a toxic relationship because you fear being alone, feel guilty about ending it, or dislike confrontation. This will only increase your risk for engaging in unhealthy behaviors, such as drinking too much, eating too much, or spending too much to "get through it."

As for the relationships that are going well, make sure that you're deliberate about taking time to be with these people, even if that means leaving work early or putting off household chores. It's usually more meaningful to share a meal, go to a movie, or watch a sunset with others than to experience it by yourself. Common sense and research show that the pursuit of happiness through healthy connections with others is *critical* for sustained well-being.

Be Kind to Others

Mark Twain once said, "The best way to cheer yourself up is to try to cheer somebody else up." Experts have found that kindness results in a surge of dopamine, the brain chemical that's involved in reward, which helps you feel good. Emory University researchers discovered that helping others triggers the same areas of the brain that turn on when people receive rewards or experience pleasure. The bottom line: Helping others brings the same pleasure we get from gratification of personal desire.

Fortunately, there are so many opportunities in everyday life to be kind, you don't have to work very hard to find them. Often, we think we have to do something dramatic to make a difference in the life of another person, but even the smallest acts of kindness can go a long way toward making you feel good, too. For instance, you can donate clothes to the Salvation Army, volunteer at a soup kitchen, or give money or time to charity. And don't forget the value of being kind to those you interact with every day.

Holding the door for someone who lives in your apartment building, giving up that prime parking spot to a mom who has a car full of young kids, even smiling at or saying hello to people you pass in the lobby on the way up to the office are all great opportunities to be considerate of others.

I had the following experiences a short time ago that demonstrated the magic of kindness and compassion toward others. I was standing in the checkout lane at the grocery store. It was snowing outside, and the woman in front of me was holding a young baby and searching through her purse to find her wallet to pay for milk and bread. She couldn't find it and said she would go home and get it. Remembering what it was like as a young mother—I always seemed to leave something behind when I went shopping with kids—I paid for her two items. She was thankful, and I felt good. And acts of kindness only seem to breed more kindness. Case in point: The next day, I was standing in the checkout line at a department store, and the woman behind me had an extra coupon for 30 percent off all purchases. When the cashier asked if I had any coupons, the woman behind me said, "You can use this." I used it and saved sixty dollars! I thanked her, and I could tell she felt good about helping me. Both giving *and* receiving left me feeling good, lifted my mood, and helped me feel more hopeful and connected to others.

Set Meaningful Goals

Most of us are busy with the demands of our daily lives and forget to stop, take a break, and look at the larger picture: What are my values? Does the way I spend my time reflect what's most important to me? What do I hope to accomplish in my life? Unfortunately, sometimes it takes an extraordinary event, such as a life-threatening illness or the loss of a loved one, to focus our attention on the meaning of life.

I urge you not to wait for these types of moments to set meaningful goals for yourself, but to make this a normal part of your everyday life. *And more important, I encourage you to try to enjoy the day-to-day process of reaching them.*

What qualifies as a meaningful goal? It depends on the individual, but, in general,

MORE THAN "JUST A MOM"

Shannon Walker, a thirty-three-year-old stay-at-home mother, sought treatment because she gained 45 pounds with her third child, had gestational diabetes during her pregnancy, and couldn't find the energy to exercise and eat healthfully to get back to her prepregnancy weight.

After the birth of her first daughter, Shannon had made the decision to leave work and stay home to raise her children. Shannon's own mother had a successful career in real estate and was never home when Shannon was growing up. She had missed her mother as a child and did not feel connected to her as an adult. Because of this, she really wanted to spend time with her children when they were young. But now, despite being happily married with three healthy kids, and active at their schools and in the community, she felt down and was increasingly gaining weight. She felt inferior to her neighbors, most of whom worked outside the home.

In her first session, she told me, "I don't work. I'm just a stay-at-home mom." I challenged her statement that she didn't work. Most mothers work 24/7 taking care of their families. I encouraged her to write about why she wanted to be home with her kids and her goals as a mother. I asked her to tell me each week how she was reaching these goals. For instance, she had potty trained her son and enabled her oldest daughter to complete her homework by herself, she wrote the monthly issue of the PTA newsletter, and so on.

Eventually Shannon began to recognize all the things she did as a mother and felt proud. She realized that she no longer needed to compare herself with others, and that accepting and appreciating her life as it was made her happy. Her choice to stay home reflected her most important values, and she learned to honor all of the good she did for her family. As her mood lifted, she started walking again each morning and eating healthfully, and the weight started to come off.

the goal must be important to you, engage your strengths and talents, and contribute to a higher purpose. Setting a goal that may be important to someone else—say your spouse or a friend—but holds little value to you won't help. Internally motivated and directed goals allow you to focus your time and energy productively. For example, you may decide to go back to college to get your teaching degree during midlife. You're not making this decision because your spouse is embarrassed by your lack of a college degree; rather, you've always wanted to be a teacher, your children are all grown up, and you now have the time and money to go back to school. You will probably be a great student, working hard and persevering through the tough classes, because getting your degree and becoming a teacher is important to you.

The same guidelines that work for setting a weight loss or exercise goal also apply to setting life goals. That is, your goals should be practical and attainable. And they should fit your talents. Otherwise your chances of success are limited. For example, setting a goal to open your own restaurant when you don't have money or practical skills isn't feasible: it'll likely lead to more frustration than satisfaction. On the other hand, working hard to achieve something that plays to your strengths and is important to you—something that reflects your true self and the source of your true passions—leads to personal satisfaction and a sense of accomplishment.

Forgive and Let Go

Is a lot of your energy focused on anger and resentment about things that happened in the past? Are you unhappy most of the time because your bitterness and hostility take up too much space in your psyche? Do these negative feelings interfere with your ability to enjoy your current blessings? Do you at times overeat to numb these feelings?

The simple fact is that life isn't fair. Every one of us must deal with life's trials and tribulations, even if you feel that you've been unfairly victimized, mistreated, abused, or neglected by others in the past. Your husband may have had an affair, your father may have been an alcoholic, you may have lost your mother at an early age, or a friend

MAKING PEACE WITH AN ALCOHOLIC MOTHER

Beth Levy, a thirty-five-year-old single woman who worked at a popular local restaurant, sought treatment for binge eating. She tended to eat healthfully all day, but she would binge when she was alone at night, especially after a shift at work.

Beth shared that she had been raised by an alcoholic mother who functioned well during the day but drank all evening. Beth often felt "trapped" by her mother, who would become sloppy as she got increasingly intoxicated. For instance, as a teenager, Beth frequently feared that her mother, who also smoked, would drop a cigarette while drunk, start a fire, and burn down the house. So Beth begrudgingly listened to her drunken mother talk about the same things night after night until she fell asleep, when Beth could be sure they were safe.

As an adult, Beth moved hundreds of miles away from her mother and rarely spoke to her. After better understanding how her mother's alcoholism had affected her, Beth realized the role her mother played in her problems, including overeating and a fear of intimacy. During treatment, Beth began to take control of her bingeing, but she still wasn't able to let go of her anger and allow others to get close to her—and I knew things wouldn't change for her until she forgave her mother.

Beth and I planned to call her mother together during several of our therapy sessions. During these conference calls, Beth was able to share with her mother the ways in which her mother's drinking had affected her ability to develop close relationships with friends, and had triggered sleep problems and an eating disorder. Her mother revealed how sad and regretful she was that she'd done to Beth what she had vowed to never do: drink too much as a mother, just as her own mother had done. They talked about the similarities in their behaviors and the ways they could support each other in recovery. They agreed to talk once a week on Sunday evenings.

Beth eventually forgave her mother, and realized that her mother—a single parent and the daughter of an alcoholic mother herself—had done the best that she could. Although her mother did not make as much progress as Beth did, they remain connected through weekly phone calls. Forgiving her mother freed up Beth's energy to pursue healthier, more meaningful connections with others.

may have betrayed your trust—any number of things can hurt or damage you. You can let yourself get stuck in those feelings by overeating or drinking too much, by sitting in front of the TV for hours at a time, or by acting out in a number of other ways. But refusing to address or resolve the source of pain, to expel the ache, and to allow for needed healing only deepens those negative emotions.

If you have let yourself get hung up on a past hurt, ask yourself: Is it painful to be stuck in this way? Is your overeating and unhappiness a result of an unresolved emotional wound? Are you perpetuating the damage by self-inflicted maltreatment? And this is crucial: At the end of the day, who is hurting? Most likely, *you* are, not the person who mistreated you. To be truly happy, you're going to have to work to get past the hurt, bitterness, and hostility. Allow yourself to be free of the past and enjoy the present. Forgiving and letting go benefits you at least as much as—and typically more than—everyone else.

Develop an Attitude of Gratitude

Learning to appreciate yourself and others is a key to a happier life. You can enjoy a heightened sense of well-being by noticing and being thankful for the blessings of everyday life—both big, such as the health of your children or the beauty of nature, and small, like the wagging tail of your beloved pet.

You develop an attitude of gratitude when you stay focused on the good things that can easily be forgotten in the business of day-to-day living. You remember to acknowledge what you have instead of what you don't. You realize that most of the positive things in your life are the ones that are consistent, such as a healthy family and friends, while the negatives usually come and go.

If you've struggled to see the bright side of situations and to be grateful for the good things in your life, it can help to keep a gratitude journal or write a gratitude letter. Try one or both of the following exercises to learn how to better recognize and appreciate the positives in your life.

Keep a Gratitude Journal Write down two things that you are grateful for each day. It's okay to repeat yourself from one day to the next. For example, you might write that you are thankful for your job and your pets every day. Or you might find different things to write about: Perhaps you feel grateful after a terrific concert and when your kids made you a great birthday card. It's so important to invest in yourself by looking at all the small things that are a source of happiness each day, and that's the whole point of this exercise: Keeping track and being mindful of daily gratitudes will help you feel better about yourself and your life.

Write a Gratitude Letter Think of someone in your life who has been especially kind or nurturing to you—someone who played an important role in your life. It could be a parent, professor, coach, or friend. Write this person a letter, be specific about how he or she helped, and express your thanks for the support. You can mail it and call to talk to the person after he or she receives it. Or the two of you can meet, and you can read the letter in person. You will feel great, and the receiver of the letter will be full of joy!

Make Time for Pleasurable Activities

Spending my professional career helping individuals overcome eating disorders has taught me many important lessons, and one that has always stuck with me is that you don't have to live a lifestyle based on deprivation to be healthy. People are inherently sensory, pleasure-seeking beings who need a certain amount of satisfaction in their lives to survive. (We discussed this in detail earlier in the book.) From infancy, we love the taste of sweet and dislike the taste of bitter. When pleasure sources are lacking, eating high-calorie, tasty foods can become a person's alternative means of enjoyment, but that can lead to obvious problems.

The brain is networked with what scientists call reward pathways and reward centers, as we've described earlier in the book. When we engage in stimulating activities that we experience as pleasurable—whether that be a delicious pizza, beautiful music, or a loving touch—these pathways trigger the release of endorphins, a type of neurotransmitter associated with positive emotion. The proper balance and interaction of these substances help to create the biochemical and psychosocial conditions that support well-being and help counter the effects of stress.

But when you don't have enough healthy sources of pleasure in your daily life, you don't experience a cascade of positive neurochemicals, thus resulting in a "reward deficiency," which in turn may trigger a state of depression or anxiety. These negative states may make you more inclined to seek out self-comforting and pain-avoidant behaviors, potentially leading to harmful addictions, cravings, and compulsions.

Unfortunately, many people simply don't make the time for pleasurable activities. The foundation of our country was built upon Puritan religious principles, which as-

THE PLEASURE OF PIZZA

Eddy Tortora, a forty-two-year-old construction worker who struggled with obesity for most of his life, grew up in an Italian household where food took center stage. He talked about how his family celebrated, mourned, and rewarded with food. Coming from an impoverished immigrant family, food was a gratifying resource—and the glue that held the family together. He described the pleasure that eating pizza gave him, even though he knew that eating this way led to weight gain.

"There is nothing like New York–style pizza after an exhausting day of work," he says. "I go to my favorite pizza joint, order mine with pepperoni, and sit in anticipation of my favorite food. I can't wait to munch on the thick crust flavored with garlic and herb seasonings, sweet tomato sauce, and extra mozzarella cheese with a hint of provolone. I'd rather enjoy a pizza over anything else." In fact, Eddy's love of pizza began to rule his life, so much that it took the place of other pleasurable experiences, like going out with friends. I worked with Eddy to help him realize the trouble his affinity for pizza could cause him if he didn't make a change. And we also worked on coming up with a list of other enjoyable activities he could engage in whenever he was tempted to turn to pizza.

sociate pleasure with sin and equate virtue with self-denial. Even today, many people feel guilty about devoting attention and energy to pleasurable pursuits and consider them a waste of time or selfish and shallow. Instead we feel we are valuable only when we are productive, multitasking, and busy every minute. With all the new technology, we are more productive but less joyful and connected with others. Many people are pushing themselves constantly and are wound up so tightly that they cannot let go and have fun.

All this pressure—pushing ourselves at home and work—whether to just get by or to pursue a higher level of success, can lead to cravings for short-term pleasure as a distraction and reward. That's why it's important to make healthy, pleasurable activities an everyday habit.

Pleasure File There are countless ways to stimulate the brain's pleasure centers. That's a good enough reason as any to go out and try something new. Leaving your comfort zone can be exciting and joyful, and it's also a great way to meet new people, which can further increase happiness. Of course, you don't have to do something new or different—you could always return to activities you haven't tried in a while. Figure out what pleasures and passions you want to pursue using the questions below.

1. What did you enjoy doing when you were younger? Did you like to read, paint, play the drums, hike, dance, listen to music, hang out with friends? Often the things that gave you pleasure as a child can offer clues about what you might enjoy now as an adult. So if you liked music when you were younger, you could look into taking piano or guitar lessons now. Or perhaps you could buy season tickets to the symphony or a nearby concert hall. If hiking was one of your favorite pastimes, get out there and find some nearby hiking trails.

2. What do you wish you had more time to do? Shop antique stores, read best sellers, travel, learn aromatherapy, play with your grandchildren, fall asleep on a ham-

mock, and so on? How can you carve out time each day to engage in one of these activities? Look at your schedule and set aside some time each day to take a step closer to making these dreams become reality.

3. Which activities so fully engage you that you lose track of time (crafting, doing yoga, making love)? Activities that require your complete attention challenge and stimulate you, but they also allow you to make satisfying progress even if the goal isn't particularly important. Examples include writing in your journal, gardening, gazing at the sunset while listening to beautiful music. Create a list of activities that fit this description.

4. Keep track of your favorite daily moments, describing in a journal the pleasure they bring you. Be specific, and focus on your five senses. For example: walking outside and feeling the warmth of the spring sun, watching your favorite sports team play, going out dancing with friends, meditating before going to work, sending a card to a friend whose mother is ill, smelling flowers or fresh-brewed coffee, listening to your favorite music, enjoying the radiant smile of a loved one. Make sure to focus on how the specific activity makes you feel and highlight the ones that bring you the most happiness.

5. Who or what makes you smile or laugh on a regular basis? Your children, favorite TV show or comedian, yourself? Receiving a witty email or sending one? Remember, you, your family, and workplace are the best sitcom—you must be willing to laugh at yourself and together with those around you. Laughing is contagious, and it's an easy way to bring in more happiness.

6. How often do you experience a warm and loving touch from another? A gentle caress, loving embrace, encouraging tap? The tactile pleasures of sex, petting your purring cat, rocking a baby to sleep, the luxury of a deep tissue massage? The sense of touch makes us feel connected and even causes the body to release brain chemicals like serotonin, resulting in your feeling more relaxed and content.

After answering these questions, make a list of all the experiences you would like to have more often. Then start a folder and collect information about hobbies, travel, opportunities for volunteering, upcoming athletic and art events, and so on. Keep the list and folder in a prominent place so that you see it every day. And most important, put the list into play: Set aside a specific time each day to do the things you love, even if it's just for five or ten minutes.

RESHAPING YOUR BRAIN

It was once believed—not too long ago, in fact—that the brain developed throughout childhood and then became immutable. With the recent advances of neuroimaging techniques such as MRI and PET scans, we now know that this is not true. Scientists have discovered that the brain has dynamic properties throughout life; that is, nerve cells (neurons) are able to form new connections, stimulate new pathways through the brain, and assume new roles and functions. In other words, our brains are evolving all the time. Through purposeful attention, mental training, and practice, we can change our brains and change ourselves. The more you practice a new behavior, the more integrated or groomed the pathway becomes. For example, research shows that meditation alters the physical structure of the brain. Brain scans reveal that experienced meditators show increased thickness in parts of the brain related to attention and sensory input. These findings are consistent with other studies that demonstrate increased thickness of music areas in the brains of musicians, and visual and motor areas in the brains of jugglers. You too can change your brain and your habits for good by following the strategies shared throughout the book.

I want to impart one important lesson: You may have been taught that you can't engage in activities you love until you finish your obligations. But you have to treat finding pleasure like you would any other must on your to-do list. If you didn't do this, it's likely that you'd never have a chance to play with your kids, read a great novel, or engage in any leisurely activities. You may even be depriving yourself of perfectly good pleasures like companionship because of this mind-set. You may be creating a state of reward deficiency, which leaves you feeling dissatisfied and anxious. To escape these feelings, you may find yourself obsessed with overindulging in delicious foods, and eventually gaining unwanted weight.

That's why I encourage you to be deliberate about engaging in activities that make you feel good and bring you joy, and expanding your pleasure file to create a more meaningful and happy life. Make time each day to take short breaks to refresh and boost your energy. Take a walk outside, get some sun, walk up and down the stairs for ten minutes at work, stretch, find a funny clip on YouTube, or use music to trigger those feel-good chemicals in your brain. These practices aren't limited to temporary well-being; they have been shown to decrease symptoms of depression and are necessary for long-term health and happiness.

PRIORITIZING YOUR HAPPINESS

The explosion of research in the field of positive psychology over the last two decades has debunked many myths about happiness. For example, we now know that the notion that people are born either happy or not happy is false. We've also learned that happiness cannot be gained through circumstantial changes, such as winning the lottery or getting married. Instead research shows that a large part of happiness is determined by what people do and how they think. This means that you're in the driver's seat.

So it's time to take your physical health and psychological well-being seriously. After reading this book, we hope you've found the motivation to make the commitment to move ahead on this journey, the courage to leave the safety of the old and pursue the new, and the ability to prioritize your quest not only for a healthy lifestyle but for happiness, too. This journey toward your goals is an amazing source of fulfillment and happiness that many people overlook or fail to pursue. The goal is not to be happy once you drop a specific number of pounds or maintain a weight for a certain time, but in pursuing these goals. Once you make the pursuit of happiness your primary goal, all of these other things will fall into place. And, hopefully, you'll soon find that with minimal effort, you can live an inspired, motivated, happy, and fulfilled life—the life you were meant to live.

Appendix 1

THE LIFESTYLE LOG

RECORDING YOUR FOOD INTAKE, exercise, and hours of sleep, as well as your emotions, moods, or situations throughout the day, offers a goldmine of information that you can use to start changing habits. You might discover that you get a lot more exercise after a good night's sleep, that you tend to chow down on cookies in the evenings after a particularly stressful day, or that your little candy nibbling habit really adds up over the course of the day. In chapters 2, 3, and 4, we ask you to use this food log for just those sorts of discoveries.

Here are a few tips on using the log:

- You can download this log for free by going to www.thebestlife.com/motivation.

- **Recording food intake.** People tend to underreport their intake by about 30 percent. In order to get the most accurate reading, write down what you eat immediately after eating. The longer you wait, the more distorted your memory. Carry blank logs with you, or write down the headings in this log on a small notebook that you carry around or even on your smartphone. Remember to record *every morsel* and *every sip*—it all counts. Also useful: snapping before and after photos of your meal, snack, or treat.

- **Recording hunger.** Using the Hunger Scale below, write down your hunger level right before and right after eating any meal, snack, or treat.

- **Recording exercise.** Write down the minutes of aerobic exercise and, using the Perceived Exertion Scale on pages 158–160, estimate your level. If you're weight training, record the number of sets and reps for each exercise as well as the weight. You can look back at old logs and see how you're progressing. If you use a pedometer, record steps but don't "double dip" by recording both steps and minutes!

- **Recording sleep.** Make a note of what time you went to bed and what time you got up, so that you can calculate how many hours of sleep you're getting each night. Write the number of hours in your log.

- **Recording situations and emotions.** Here's where you jot down "Stressed at work trying to meet a deadline," or "Angry because _____ criticized me," or "Tired," or any other mood state or situation.

The Hunger Scale

Sometimes it's not easy to determine if your desire to eat is driven by true physical hunger, emotions, or the brain wiring described in chapter 3. But learning to eat only when you're actually hungry is key to avoiding overeating and to control your weight. The Hunger Scale will help you do just that.

Here's how it works: Before you start eating a meal or snack, rate your hunger level using the scale on the following page and record it in the Lifestyle Log. Ideally, you should eat when you're at a level 3 or 4. Try not to let yourself get to a 1 or 2; at these levels, you're

LIFESTYLE LOG

TIME OF DAY	SLEEP (NUMBER OF HOURS)	HUNGER SCALE; BEFORE AND AFTER EATING (I.E., 3/6)	FOOD AND DRINK (LIST SPECIFIC AMOUNTS)	EXERCISE (TYPE, MINUTES OR STEPS, PERCEIVED EXERTION)	SITUATION/EMOTIONS (I.E., IN THE KITCHEN, STRESSED AT WORK, BORED AT HOME)

more likely to overdo it. After a meal, jot down your hunger level again; you should aim to stop eating when you reach 5 (the level recommended for weight loss). Later, after you've hit your goal weight, you can stop eating at 6 (the level recommended for maintenance).

10   Stuffed. You are so full, you feel nauseated.

9   Very uncomfortably full. You need to loosen your clothes.

8   Uncomfortably full. You feel bloated.

7   Full. You feel a little bit uncomfortable.

6   Perfectly comfortable. You feel satisfied.

5   Comfortable. You're more or less satisfied but could eat a little more.

4   Slightly uncomfortable. You're just beginning to feel signs of hunger.

3   Uncomfortable. Your stomach is rumbling.

2   Very uncomfortable. You feel irritable and unable to concentrate.

1   Weak and light-headed. Your stomach acid is churning.

Appendix 2

BODY MASS INDEX

WHEN IT COMES TO body weight, what matters more than the number on the scale is how much of that weight is muscle (lean tissue) and how much is fat. Scientists devised a formula, which in many cases correlates pretty closely with body fat in adults: the body mass index (BMI). BMI is basically a ratio of height to weight, and the BMI scale is the basis for terms such as *overweight* and *obesity*. These are the widely accepted BMI categories:

Underweight: BMI 18.5 or under
Normal weight: BMI 18.6 to 24.9 (18.6 to 22.9 for Asians*)
Overweight: BMI 25 to 29.5 (23 to 26.9 for Asians)
Obese: 30 or higher (27 or higher for Asians)

The overweight category is associated with an increased risk for heart disease, diabetes, and cancer. In some studies, a BMI in this range correlates to a percent body fat of 32

---

* The BMI cutoffs for Asians are different because, at the same BMI number, Asians typically carry more fat than African Americans, Hispanics, or white Americans.

percent to 36 percent for women and 20 percent to 25 percent for men. Body fat exceeding 30 percent for women and 25 percent for men is considered risky.

The obese category is associated with an even greater risk for the same conditions mentioned above. Some studies indicate that a BMI of 30 correlates to a percent body fat of 39 percent to 42 percent for women and 25 percent to 30 percent for men.

The BMI isn't a foolproof assessment of body fat and, therefore, of health risk. For instance, because the BMI formula is based on weight and height, heavy but muscular people with low levels of body fat can fall into the overweight or obese categories. Many football players and bodybuilders have BMIs of 25 or more but have a low percentage of body fat. On the flip side, some people, particularly the elderly, who have little muscle mass, may have a BMI in the "normal" range but actually have a high percentage of body fat.

And BMI doesn't reflect the *distribution* of your body fat. And that makes a big health difference. If much of your fat is concentrated deep in your belly (visceral fat), you're at a greater risk for heart disease, cancer, and diabetes. But if it's mainly sitting on your hips and thighs, it poses little to no risk. A waistline of more than 35 inches for women (31½ for Asian women) and 40 inches for men (35½ for Asian men) is considered risky. (To measure, place the tape around the largest part of your belly.)

Look for your BMI on the following chart or get it automatically calculated by going to www.thebestlife.com/motivation. If you're curious and want to calculate it yourself, the formula is:

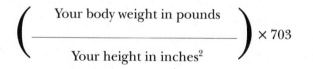

$$\left(\frac{\text{Your body weight in pounds}}{\text{Your height in inches}^2} \right) \times 703$$

BMI	Normal						Overweight					Obese					
	19	20	21	22	23	24	25	26	27	28	29	30	31	32	33	34	35
Height (inches)																	
58	91	96	100	105	110	115	119	124	129	134	138	143	148	153	158	162	167
59	94	99	104	109	114	119	124	128	133	138	143	148	153	158	163	168	173
60	97	102	107	112	118	123	128	133	138	143	148	153	158	163	168	174	179
61	100	106	111	116	122	127	132	137	143	148	153	158	164	169	174	180	185
62	104	109	115	120	126	131	136	142	147	153	158	164	169	175	180	186	191
63	107	113	118	124	130	135	141	146	152	158	163	169	175	180	186	191	197
64	110	116	122	128	134	140	145	151	157	163	169	174	180	186	192	197	204
65	114	120	126	132	138	144	150	156	162	168	174	180	186	192	198	204	210
66	118	124	130	136	142	148	155	161	167	173	179	186	192	198	204	210	216
67	121	127	134	140	146	153	159	166	172	178	185	191	198	204	211	217	223
68	125	131	138	144	151	158	164	171	177	184	190	197	203	210	216	223	230
69	128	135	142	149	155	162	169	176	182	189	196	203	209	216	223	230	236
70	132	139	146	153	160	167	174	181	188	195	202	209	216	222	229	236	243
71	136	143	150	157	165	172	179	186	193	200	208	215	222	229	236	243	250
72	140	147	154	162	169	177	184	191	199	206	213	221	228	235	242	250	258
73	144	151	159	166	174	182	189	197	204	212	219	227	235	242	250	257	265
74	148	155	163	171	179	186	194	202	210	218	225	233	241	249	256	264	272
75	152	160	168	176	184	192	200	208	216	224	232	240	248	256	264	272	279
76	156	164	172	180	189	197	205	213	221	230	238	246	254	263	271	279	287

Source: Adapted from *Clinical Guidelines on the Identification, Evaluation, and Treatment of Overweight and Obesity in Adults: The Evidence Report.*

Index Table

				Extreme Obesity														
36	37	38	39	40	41	42	43	44	45	46	47	48	49	50	51	52	53	54

Body Weight (pounds)

36	37	38	39	40	41	42	43	44	45	46	47	48	49	50	51	52	53	54
172	177	181	186	191	196	201	205	210	215	220	224	229	234	239	244	248	253	258
178	183	188	193	198	203	208	212	217	222	227	232	237	242	247	252	257	262	267
184	189	194	199	204	209	215	220	225	230	235	240	245	250	255	261	266	271	276
190	195	201	206	211	217	222	227	232	238	243	248	254	259	264	269	275	280	285
196	202	207	213	218	224	229	235	240	246	251	256	262	267	273	278	284	289	295
203	208	214	220	225	231	237	242	248	254	259	265	270	278	282	287	293	299	304
209	215	221	227	232	238	244	250	256	262	267	273	279	285	291	296	302	308	314
216	222	228	234	240	246	252	258	264	270	276	282	288	294	300	306	312	318	324
223	229	235	241	247	253	260	266	272	278	284	291	297	303	309	315	322	328	334
230	236	242	249	255	261	268	274	280	287	293	299	306	312	319	325	331	338	344
236	243	249	256	262	269	276	282	289	295	302	308	315	322	328	335	341	348	354
243	250	257	263	270	277	284	291	297	304	311	318	324	331	338	345	351	358	365
250	257	264	271	278	285	292	299	306	313	320	327	334	341	348	355	362	369	376
257	265	272	279	286	293	301	308	315	322	329	338	343	351	358	365	372	379	386
265	272	279	287	294	302	309	316	324	331	338	346	353	361	368	375	383	390	397
272	280	288	295	302	310	318	325	333	340	348	355	363	371	378	386	393	401	408
280	287	295	303	311	319	326	334	342	350	358	365	373	381	389	396	404	412	420
287	295	303	311	319	327	335	343	351	359	367	375	383	391	399	407	415	423	431
295	304	312	320	328	336	344	353	361	369	377	385	394	402	410	418	426	435	443

Appendix 3

THE GOLDBERG DEPRESSION SCALE

Use this questionnaire to help determine whether you should see a mental health professional for diagnosis and treatment of depression, or to monitor your mood.

You might reproduce this scale and use it on a weekly basis to track your moods. It also might be used to show your doctor how your symptoms have changed from one visit to the next. Changes of five or more points are significant. This scale is not designed to make a diagnosis of depression or take the place of a professional diagnosis. If you suspect that you are depressed, please consult with a mental health professional as soon as possible.

The eighteen statements on the following pages refer to how you have felt and behaved during the past week. For each item, indicate the extent to which it is true by circling the appropriate number below the statement.

1. I do things slowly.

(0) Not at all
(1) Just a little
(2) Somewhat
(3) Moderately
(4) Quite a lot
(5) Very much

2. My future seems hopeless.

(0) Not at all
(1) Just a little
(2) Somewhat
(3) Moderately
(4) Quite a lot
(5) Very much

3. It is hard for me to concentrate on reading.

(0) Not at all
(1) Just a little
(2) Somewhat
(3) Moderately
(4) Quite a lot
(5) Very much

4. The pleasure and joy have gone out of my life.

(0) Not at all
(1) Just a little
(2) Somewhat
(3) Moderately
(4) Quite a lot
(5) Very much

5. I have difficulty making decisions.

(0) Not at all
(1) Just a little
(2) Somewhat
(3) Moderately
(4) Quite a lot
(5) Very much

6. I have lost interest in aspects of my life that used to be important to me.

(0) Not at all
(1) Just a little
(2) Somewhat
(3) Moderately
(4) Quite a lot
(5) Very much

7. I feel sad, blue, and unhappy.

(0) Not at all

(1) Just a little

(2) Somewhat

(3) Moderately

(4) Quite a lot

(5) Very much

8. I am agitated and keep moving around.

(0) Not at all

(1) Just a little

(2) Somewhat

(3) Moderately

(4) Quite a lot

(5) Very much

9. I feel fatigued.

(0) Not at all

(1) Just a little

(2) Somewhat

(3) Moderately

(4) Quite a lot

(5) Very much

10. It takes great effort for me to do simple things.

(0) Not at all

(1) Just a little

(2) Somewhat

(3) Moderately

(4) Quite a lot

(5) Very much

11. I feel that I am a guilty person who deserves to be punished.

(0) Not at all

(1) Just a little

(2) Somewhat

(3) Moderately

(4) Quite a lot

(5) Very much

12. I feel like a failure.

(0) Not at all

(1) Just a little

(2) Somewhat

(3) Moderately

(4) Quite a lot

(5) Very much

13. I feel lifeless—more dead than alive.

(0) Not at all
(1) Just a little
(2) Somewhat
(3) Moderately
(4) Quite a lot
(5) Very much

14. I'm getting too much, too little, or not enough restful sleep.

(0) Not at all
(1) Just a little
(2) Somewhat
(3) Moderately
(4) Quite a lot
(5) Very much

15. I spend time thinking about HOW I might kill myself.

(0) Not at all
(1) Just a little
(2) Somewhat
(3) Moderately
(4) Quite a lot
(5) Very much

16. I feel trapped or caught.

(0) Not at all
(1) Just a little
(2) Somewhat
(3) Moderately
(4) Quite a lot
(5) Very much

17. I feel depressed even when good things happen to me.

(0) Not at all
(1) Just a little
(2) Somewhat
(3) Moderately
(4) Quite a lot
(5) Very much

18. Without trying to diet, I have lost or gained weight.

(0) Not at all
(1) Just a little
(2) Somewhat
(3) Moderately
(4) Quite a lot
(5) Very much

Score Interpretation

Add up your total points. The higher the number, the more severe your depression may be. If you take the quiz again weekly or monthly, changes of 5 or more points between tests may be significant. Use the ranges below as a guide.

Score ranges:

0–9 no depression likely

10–17 possibly mildly depressed

18–21 borderline depression

22–35 mild to moderate depression

36–53 moderate to severe depression

54 and up severely depressed

GOAL-SETTING WORKSHEET

AS YOU WORK ON changing habits, you need to set goals, such as going out for a walk five days a week, or limiting sweets to 150 calories per day, or setting aside thirty relaxing minutes for yourself each day. The goal-setting worksheet on the next page (first described on page 78) will help ensure that your goals really happen. It helps you set realistic, manageable, and very specific goals. Toward the end of chapters 2, 3, and 4, we've filled in examples for you. It might help to refer back to them before you use this blank worksheet to set your own goal. You may use this again and again for all your various goals. You can print out a free copy of this worksheet at www.thebestlife.com/motivation.

Use the worksheet to set a goal that you can and will work on during the next twenty-four hours. The next day, after you've tried out your strategy, set a two-week goal, which is short enough not to be overwhelming but long enough to start setting up a good habit. Revisit your plan in two weeks. If it's still working and it's the most you can do (let's say that you are exercising an hour in the morning on Monday and Friday), then stick with it. If the plan isn't working well or you can do even more (exercise three days a week instead of two), then adjust your plan.

1. What is my goal?

   Find a goal that you *know* you can achieve—nothing overly ambitious.

2. What is the most positive outcome of achieving this goal?

   This is crucial: You *must* be able to name and imagine a benefit. Otherwise, this technique won't work; the positive outcome is what's driving motivation and infusing meaning.

3. What is the main obstacle standing in my way?

4. How can I overcome the obstacle?

   Be very specific, noting when and where the obstacle occurs.

5. How do I prevent the obstacle from occurring in the first place?

   Again, be specific about when and where.

6. How, specifically, should I achieve my goal?

   For this answer, focus specifically when and where you can make it happen; for example: "Get to the park by 7 a.m. on Monday, Wednesday, and Friday to power walk for 45 minutes."

Appendix 5

THE MOTIVATIONAL INTERVIEW

HOW MOTIVATED—AND READY—ARE YOU to make healthy lifestyle changes? The motivational interview will help answer those questions. It will also help guide you to the specific changes you're most ready to make. The motivational interview was first used to help people break their addiction to alcohol or drugs and is now being used successfully to help motivate people to make diet and exercise changes.

You first saw this interview in chapter 2, where it was used to help you overcome emotional eating. In chapters 3 and 4, we suggested that you flip to this appendix and take the motivational interview again, this time directed at either eating a healthier diet or increasing exercise.

Traditionally, a therapist asks the question and the patient responds. In this case, you're going to be both the therapist *and* the patient. As therapist, you'll be compassionate and nonjudgmental—no putting yourself down! The goal isn't to make yourself feel guilty, it's to know yourself better. For instance, instead of saying, "Why are you killing yourself with all that junk food?" which is bound to shut you right down, ask yourself how your eating habits are affecting your life. A much more thoughtful, helpful answer will come out of that question. It's quite possible to have thoughts and feelings that you suppress, and you won't realize what they are until you let them bubble to the surface. This is your chance to be introspective, prodded by the questions that your therapist (aka you) is going to ask.

As the "patient," you'll need to look deep within yourself to honestly answer the questions and take responsibility for your responses—even (and especially) if you don't like what you hear. You may, for instance, not like to admit to yourself that you gave up swimming, the only type of exercise you really like, because you felt embarrassed walking from the locker room to the pool in a bathing suit. Or that you don't want to give up your junk food habit because, despite the heartache it's causing, you really enjoy the high you get from food.

In your role as the therapist, you'll need to draw the truth out of yourself, and note where there's resistance to change ("I have to be there to wake my kids up in the morning"), and prompt your patient to look for a way to resolve the resistance ("Well, actually, maybe my husband could hold down the fort until I get back from the gym").

Take your time with the motivational interview. Write down your answers; they'll serve as a reference point to how you're progressing, and some of them will offer you a motivating reminder during those times when your enthusiasm wanes. Use this interview for any healthy lifestyle change you want to make. Tailor it to your needs by filling in the blanks. In parentheses, we've offered an exercise or diet suggestion. Now pull out a pad of paper and get comfortable.

ARE YOU MOTIVATED? GAUGE HOW MUCH

1. How is my current weight affecting my life right now?

2. How is _____ (not getting enough exercise or an unhealthy diet) affecting my life right now?

3. On a scale of 0 to 10 (with 0 being not at all important and 10 being critically important), how important is it for me to _____ (get more exercise or improve my eating habits)?

4. What kinds of things have I done in the past to _____ (start exercising or eat healthier)?

5. Which of these strategies worked and which strategies didn't? Why?

6. Some people say that they're divided: They want to _____ (get enough exercise or eat healthier), but part of them doesn't really want to change. Is this at all true for me?

7. On a scale of 0 to 10 (with 0 being not ready at all and 10 being very ready), how ready am I to work on _____ (getting enough exercise, such as setting aside time to work out, or eating healthier, such as stocking my kitchen with healthy foods)?

8. What could I start doing today or tomorrow to overcome _____ (my exercise resistance or junk food habit)?

9. What was my life like before I _____ (became so sedentary or started overeating)?

10. How much does it worry me that I might return to old patterns of _____ (being sedentary or not getting enough exercise or overeating) once I change them?

11. What makes me feel like I can sustain my progress?

12. What are my hopes for the future if I am able to _____ (become physically active, have a healthy diet, and/or lose some weight)?

13. How would my life be different if I _____ (started exercising, eating better, and/or lost weight and adopted a healthier lifestyle)?

Interpreting Your Answers: Exercise-Related Interview

Question 1: *How is my current weight affecting my life right now?*

There are really two ways you can go when answering this question. One is the obvious answer; the other is the deeper and more relevant answer. On the surface, maybe your response is that your weight is making you feel unattractive and even embarrassed. In short, you feel bad about yourself. This isn't to suggest that this isn't important—it is very, very important—but let's also talk about other problems that you may not want to think about as much. Maybe your weight is keeping you from fully participating in life: You don't go to parties because you think you look fat in dressier clothes. You love the beach but hate to go because putting on a bathing suit is a nightmare. You don't play on the playground with your kids because it's physically uncomfortable for you. Traveling isn't fun because you hate having to squeeze into an airline seat, and sightseeing is a drag because you have all that extra weight to haul around.

Another thing you should think about is how your weight is affecting your health. You may feel fine and even get a good report from the doctor each time you undergo a checkup. But being overweight can take a toll. It's the rare person that doesn't develop some sort of adverse health effect related to being overweight. This may not be affecting your life now, but don't ignore the fact that it could affect your life significantly in the future.

Consider the life you have now and consider the life you want to have. If they're not the same, and part of that is because you're uncomfortable with your weight, then you know you've got to make some major changes. Let regular exercise be one of those changes.

Question 2: *How is being sedentary, or not getting enough exercise, affecting my life right now?*

If you're honest, lack of exercise in your life may be kind of a plus. It gives you more time for other things, you don't have to spend any money on workout shoes or gym memberships, and you don't have to put your body through some truly uncomfortable paces. Maybe you even love the fact that you don't have to worry about having to deal with sweaty hair. So life without exercise is, well, pretty good.

On the other hand, is it really that good when you're so out of shape that walking the length of the local mall is exhausting? Is it really that good when you're cranky all the time? How about when you don't have the strength to carry groceries, do work around the house, or even hold a crying child or grandchild that needs comforting for any length of time? If there was an emergency, could you pick up that child and run? You may have more minutes in the day to devote to work or personal interests, but is it worth the risk of illnesses that could potentially take away all of your free time? I'm simply asking you to weigh the pros and cons: What are you getting in exchange for not exercising, and is it worth missing out on the benefits?

Question 3: *On a scale of 0 to 10 (with 0 being not at all important and 10 being critically important), how important is it for me to get more exercise and become more fit?*

In chapter 4 you were asked to zero in on something that you felt could help motivate you to exercise regularly. If you gave the importance of fitness a 5 or lower, then you probably still haven't found a compelling reason to be physically active. Perhaps you think that cutting calories alone will be enough for you; if that's it, go back and take a quick look at chapter 6, which describes the results of the National Weight Control Registry study. Virtually no one succeeds at weight loss without some physical activity worked into the mix.

If you gave the importance of fitness closer to a 10, then you've taken a first step toward making exercise a reality in your life. What you're going to need to work on now is how to get past the discomfort and other barriers that can keep even people who really believe activity is important from fulfilling their goals.

Questions 4 and 5: *What kinds of things have I done in the past to start exercising or to step up the pace? Which of these strategies worked and which didn't? Why?*

These questions are meant to help you assess your past experience with exercise. There are so many things that stop people from exercising, among them bad relationships and a simple inability to juggle both life's tribulations and a regular exercise schedule. Many people also give up on an exercise routine because they don't feel capable while working out. Did you always seem to get tired out (or bored) before you reached one mile? Did you feel clumsy in exercise class? Did you never seem able to lift anything but the lightest weights? It's easy to think that you're just not good at exercise—that's why you always quit—but before you come to that conclusion, think back on what *did* work, even if it happened a long time ago. Maybe it's been years since you played tennis, but you really liked it. Could you start playing again? Maybe you used to walk with your former next-door neighbor, which made it so much easier to endure—you hardly noticed the miles going by. Could you enlist someone in your new neighborhood (or seek out a walking group; even start one with colleagues during your lunch break)?

It doesn't really matter exactly what prevented you from exercising regularly in the past. What matters is that the potential for that bump in the road to derail you again has now been significantly reduced or removed. Assess your present circumstances with care. It's also important that you be ready to get creative about finding ways to sustain exercise. Most of all, don't let flashbacks of past failures hold you back. If you are motivated enough, you'll be able to keep an exercise regimen going regardless of your previous experience with activity.

Questions 6 and 7: *Some people say that they're divided—they want to get enough exercise, but part of them doesn't really want to change. Is this at all true for me? On a scale of 0 to 10 (with 0 being not ready at all and 10 being very ready), how ready am I to work on getting enough exercise, such as setting aside time to work out?*

Because exercise is an imperative in our society—everyone from the surgeon general on down recommends it—there is probably a side of you that wants to comply, to do the right thing. But you may also feel ambivalent. You don't like exercise, so deep down you don't really want to do it. Be up front about your ambivalence. If you don't admit it to yourself, you're going to repeatedly start and stop exercising, always wondering why it doesn't work out. You shouldn't start an exercise program unless you're deeply committed to it. This book is designed to help you find that level of commitment, so use the tools in the preceding pages to assist you. But don't start until you're ready to do the work.

And what does it mean to be ready to exercise? It means more than just wanting it to happen. It means that you are ready to take the time to sit down with a calendar and map out an exercise schedule. Or ready to inform your family that you are setting aside time for activity and that it's nonnegotiable. Or ready to study up on a way to properly build up your workouts so that you don't exercise so hard in the beginning that you feel terrible and quit. Be enthusiastic; yes, that's half the battle. But being ready also means being prepared to deal with the practicalities of becoming an active person.

Questions 8 to 11: *What could I start doing today or tomorrow to overcome my exercise resistance? What was my life like before I became so sedentary (or lowered my level of physical activity)? How much does it worry me that I might return to old patterns of being sedentary, or sporadic, about exercise once I change them? What makes me feel like I can sustain my progress?*

How about starting small. Take a short walk outside and see if you don't feel better when you get home. You probably will. That small effort may jog your memory. Think back on the times when you were more active. No doubt it felt good, especially if you were trimmer and stronger as a result. But even if you've never been active a day in your life (that you can remember), imagine what it could feel like in the future. Visualize feeling lighter and more energetic. Maybe you're playing outdoors with your children, or hiking in the mountains, or on vacation, walking around a new city. You've doing it with vigor and no pain, and it's immensely enjoyable. Keep these images in your head. They're going to inspire you now—and help you *stay* inspired, too.

Still, past experiences have the potential to put you off exercise. Let's amend that: past *negative* experiences. So if you're worried that you might return to your old patterns of stopping and starting exercise, approach it differently than you have before. Choose a different activity, a different time of day, a different place. Enlist a workout buddy. Be creative and flexible so that you're able to create a new pattern—one that you enjoy.

Questions 12 and 13: *What are my hopes for the future if I am able to become physically active and/or lose some weight? How would my life be different if I started exercising (or ramped up my current level) and/or lost weight and adopted a healthier lifestyle?*

Visualize yourself lighter and able to move more freely. Imagine being strong enough to lift boxes and groceries with minimal effort. Picture yourself going up stairs and chasing after a child without getting winded. These are some of the rewards of becoming a fit person. Allow these mental images to creep into your consciousness so that you can *feel* what it's like to be a regular exerciser. It's a little like practicing self-hypnosis. Letting yourself experience positive changes, if only through your imagination, can motivate you to strive to make those changes real. As you think about what the future will hold, see the life you want in front of you—then go out and make it a reality.

Interpreting Your Answers: Eating and Nutrition Interview

Questions 1 and 2: *How is my current weight affecting my life right now? How are my eating habits affecting my life right now?*

When thinking through the consequences of your current way of eating, you may have listed "high blood pressure" or "setting myself up for cancer," or any of the other diseases mentioned in the Why List starting on page 91. Or disease risk might not have even made your list when answering these questions. Instead it could be something like not being able to join your family and friends for a walk or a shopping trip because your body weight makes moving around uncomfortable. Go back to these answers when your motivation flags—it's a reminder of where you don't want to be.

Along with the negatives, don't censor yourself if some of the advantages to your current way of eating occur to you. In fact, take a few moments to think about that. Despite the heartache it's causing, you wouldn't be eating this way if there weren't some benefits. For instance, you enjoy the high you get from food. Or, after exhausting internal battles over food, such as trying to restrain yourself from opening a bag of chips, giving in is simply a big relief.

So go ahead and write down both the negative consequences and the plusses. As you work on your eating issues, you'll find that the new benefits far outweigh the old ones.

Question 3. On a scale of 0 to 10 (with 0 being not at all important and 10 being critically important), how important is it for me to change my eating habits?

As we emphasize throughout this book, motivation hinges largely on seeing that a behavior is important to you and believing you'll benefit from it. If you answered a 5 or lower on this question, then go back and reread the Why List to see if that helps bump your number up a little. The more importance you place on nutrition and on regaining control over your eating habits, the easier it's going to be for you to do just that.

Questions 4 and 5. What kinds of things have I done in the past to address my eating issues? Which of these strategies worked and which didn't? Why?

Another key to motivation is the sense that you're capable, that you feel you can handle the task at hand—in this case, changing your eating habits. In question 4, you're listing ways that you've improved your eating before; in question 5, you're narrowing it down to what actually worked, at least for a while. "Worked" means that you not only improved the nutritional quality of your diet and/or decreased cravings for unhealthy foods, but also that the habits you developed were ones that you could live with over the long haul. So many times people say they just love this diet or that diet, but talk to them a few weeks later, and they've burned out on it. "I just couldn't keep eating all that salmon" or "Too much cooking was involved—I was exhausted." But when you find some healthy cereals that you like, or you start taking a short walk at the time of day that you used to have a doughnut—and enjoy the walk—these are the successful changes that you should focus on.

What if nothing has ever worked when it comes to trying to overcome food addiction or eat a nutritious diet? Then shift to other accomplishments in your life: school- or job-related achievements, your ability to make and keep friendships, your parenting or leadership skills, or anything else you're proud of and know you're good at. Can any of those skills transfer to overcoming your diet issues? Keep in mind that if you were able to master other tasks, with the right mind-set, you can change your diet as well.

Questions 6, 7, and 8: *Some people say that they're divided—they want a nutritious diet and to feel in control around food, but part of them doesn't really want to change. Is this at all true for me? On a scale of 0 to 10 (with 0 being not ready at all and 10 being very ready), how ready am I to work on improving my diet and/or gaining control over food? For instance, am I ready to experience the momentary discomfort of not giving into a craving? What could I start doing today or tomorrow to tackle my eating issues?*

These questions reveal how ready you are to change your eating habits. Answering them honestly, it could turn out that you're not very ready or enthusiastic about it—maybe question 6 revealed some ambivalence (totally normal), or you scored, say, a 2 on question 7. That's okay—a 2 is better than a 0. And if you wrote down 0, give it a little more thought. Are you sure you're not ready to do *anything*, even something small such as adding a fruit or a vegetable to your day? If it's truly 0, then read through chapter 3 and see if you're willing to try any of the suggestions. If not, come back when you do feel more ready. Meanwhile, you might be up for making some changes on the exercise front (chapter 4) or addressing emotional issues (chapters 2, 5, and 7).

If you approach treating your food addiction (or other diet issues) smartly, with realistic goals and approaches that fit into your life, you'll usually find that after a while 2 moves up to a 3, then a 5, and so on. As you gain mastery on the food front, resistance starts melting away. In the Nine Step Program starting on page 98, we're going to help you start off on the right foot. Where to begin? Give some thought to question 8 on what you could do, and we'll offer up more ideas in chapters 2 and 3.

Questions 9, 12, and 13: *What was my life like before, when my diet was more nutritious and I felt more in charge of my food choices? What are my hopes for the future if I'm able to gain control over my diet and lose weight (if needed)? How would my life be different if I started eating a nutritious diet and lost weight (if needed)?*

Put all your fears and insecurities about changing your eating habits on hold while you answer these questions, and imagine how you'd feel if you were in control of your diet and eating healthfully. Allow yourself to relish the sensation of leaving a meal satisfied but not stuffed, of being able to put one scoop of ice cream in your bowl, enjoy it, and not feel compelled to return to the freezer the rest of the night. If you're currently overweight, picture yourself at a healthy weight, being able to walk with greater ease and more energy. These are images you can conjure up when you need a shot of motivation.

Questions 10 and 11: *How much does it worry me that I might return to old eating patterns once I change them? What makes me feel like I can sustain my progress?*

Even things that worked may not have worked for long—that's probably why you're reading this book. Question 10 gets at your fear that even if you make changes again, they may not last. If you've lost and gained back weight repeatedly, it's natural that you might not feel all that capable of sustaining a weight loss. Here's a little fact to boost your confidence: As we reported earlier in this book, 90 percent of the successful weight maintainers in the National Weight Control Registry went through cycles of weight loss and regain. The average maintainer in this study lost a mean of 565 pounds before the weight loss finally stuck.

Analyze why things have fallen apart in the past and see if you can prevent any of the forces that destabilized your diet. Maybe a major stressor hit, like a move or you lost your job. In chapter 2, you can pick up some great coping skills that will give you a better way to deal with stress next time. Or maybe you had a relapse and gave up—that's a classic. The section on black-and-white thinking featured in the Nine Step Program will help you deal differently next time.

Question 11 takes the opposite view: What are the reasons you might be more likely to sustain it this time? Maybe you feel more ready now. Or you have more experience to draw from, so you can eliminate the all-salmon diet and other unsustainable techniques and give strategies that worked another try. Many of the approaches in the Nine Step Program will resonate with you.

Appendix 6

THE BEST LIFE APPROACH TO EXERCISE

By Bob Greene

TRYING TO EXERCISE ON a catch-as-catch-can basis hardly ever works. To stay motivated and reap the many benefits of exercise, you need to exercise regularly and consistently. And to exercise regularly and consistently, you need to make fitness part of your schedule so that you do it as habitually as you, say, brush your teeth or eat lunch. You put aside time every day to do those things; now put aside time every day (or almost every day) for exercise.

The most effective fitness regimens include exercises that address three primary areas of fitness: functional fitness, cardiovascular (also known as aerobic) fitness, and strength. As I noted on pages 156–157, there are time, intensity, and frequency marks you'll need to hit in order to maximize your results from cardiovascular exercise as well as specific benchmarks for functional fitness and strength training. A good starting place is the following twelve-week cardio, strength training, and functional fitness plan. It will not only get you started, it will also give you a template for long-term fitness. (The fact that it's twelve weeks long doesn't mean it's over in twelve weeks; consider it a launching pad for ongoing exercise.) The plan is similar to the one I gave readers in *The Best Life Guide to Managing Diabetes and Pre-Diabetes*. I like it because it works for just about everyone, and it pays particular attention to the type of exercise that helps burn fat and improve blood glucose levels. Even if you don't have diabetes or prediabetes, it will give your health a boost.

The Plan, Part 1: Functional Fitness

If you haven't engaged in any significant physical activity for a long time, it's a good idea to start with functional fitness exercises: a combination of stretches and strengthening exercises that often use your own body weight for resistance. Simple, yet succinct, they better your core strength, flexibility, balance, and coordination, improving posture and helping you move more gracefully. All that is also going to make your everyday movements easier: toting groceries, lifting a suitcase, carrying a child who refuses to walk, reaching for a coat in the back of a closet—those things become less arduous when you are functionally fit.

Just as important, functional fitness exercises prepare you to perform the cardiovascular and strength-training workouts you need to both manage your weight and increase your well-being. By helping you build up strength and flexibility, they reduce your likelihood of injury when you begin those more rigorous forms of exercise, and they also make cardio and strength-training workouts feel like less of a chore. That's going to help you stick with the twelve-week program and beyond.

The functional fitness exercises that follow take so little time to perform that you could—and should—do them every day. Here are four strengtheners and seven stretches to work into your routine.

Functional Fitness Exercises

HEEL RAISE

- Standing on a board approximately 2 inches by 36 inches, or any other raised, stable surface (no more than 2 to 3 inches high), place the ball of each foot on the raised area, with heels on the floor. Keep feet about 12 inches apart; knees are straight, but not locked. Slowly raise heels as high as you can and hold for 1 second before slowly lowering down to starting position. Repeat for a total of 15 stretches.

SHRUG ROLL

- Stand up straight, feet a little apart and arms at your sides. Shrug shoulders up toward your ears as high as they can go. Pause for a second in this position, then roll shoulders back while squeezing your shoulder blades together. Pause for a second in midsqueeze, then drop shoulders back to starting position. Repeat 10 times; do two sets.

THE BASIC CRUNCH

- Lie on your back, with knees bent and heels 12 to 15 inches from your buttocks. Place both your hands behind your neck.

- Let your abs do the work of raising your torso straight up at a 30 degree to 45 degree angle, but don't curl your body or your back up. Point your chin to the ceiling.

- Hold for 1 second, then lower down. Repeat 15 times for one set.

THE TWISTING TRUNK CURL

- Lie on your back, with knees bent and heels 12 to 15 inches from your buttocks.

- Place your right ankle over your left knee.

- Place both hands behind your neck.

- Using your abs to power you, raise your right shoulder toward the left knee, just 8 to 12 inches off the ground. Then return to start position.

- Do 15 on this side, then switch legs and repeat for another 15 moves.

UPPER AB CRUNCHES

- Lie on your back with your elbows out, fingers touching the sides of your forehead.

- Bend your knees and hips until your legs are at 90 degrees; it's best to have a ball or chair support your feet.

- Raise your torso at a 35 degree to 45 degree angle and hold for a second.

- Return to start position. Perform two sets of 15 to 20 repetitions.

THE ARM AND LEG RAISE

- Lie on your stomach, arms stretched out in front of you, with your head supported by a folded towel. (The towel goes under your armpits and under your chin.)

▪ Raise your right arm and your left leg simultaneously by contracting your abdominal muscles and lower back muscles. Keep your shoulders and pelvis pressed against the floor. Meanwhile, your left arm and right leg should be on the floor.

▪ Lift to the point where you feel a gentle tension in the lower back muscles. Pause for a second before going back to starting position.

▪ Do 15 on one side, then switch so that your left arm and right leg are raised and do another 15.

LATERAL NECK STRETCH

▪ Tilt your head to the side, ear to shoulder.

▪ Hold on each side for about 15 seconds.

▪ Repeat 5 times.

MIDDLE AND LOWER BACK STRETCH

▪ Seated on a chair with your knees apart, hold your arms out in front of you and stretch. Keeping them in this position, gradually bend forward until you feel a gentle tension in your upper and/or middle back. (At this point, your arms may be between your knees, hands touching the floor if possible.) Hold the stretch for 5 seconds, relax for 5 seconds, and repeat 2 more times.

STANDING HAMSTRING STRETCH

▪ Stand with one leg up on a step or on a chair in front of you. Place hands on hips, making sure you're stable. Keep the leg that is lifted straight and slowly bend toward your toes, keeping your back straight until you feel a stretch. Hold for 5 seconds (no bouncing) and relax for another 5 seconds. Repeat on each leg 3 to 5 times.

QUADRICEPS STRETCH

- Standing, hold on to a chair back with your right hand. Use the other hand to clutch your left ankle behind you, knee bent. Bring your heel toward your buttocks until you feel a little tension in your thigh. Keep the knee of the other leg slightly bent. Both knees should be parallel. Hold for 5 seconds, relax for 5 seconds, and continue this way for 3 to 4 stretches. Repeat on the other side.

UPPER CALF STRETCH

- Standing, hold on to a chair back with your left hand while placing the other hand on your right hip. Bend your left leg about 45 degrees, keeping your left knee right above your left foot (not in front of it). Bring your right leg behind you, keeping it straight, with the heel on the floor. If you don't feel the stretch in this leg, bring the opposite (bent) leg forward a little more. Do not arch your back; hold the stretch for 5 seconds, relax for 5 seconds, repeat 2 more times. Then switch legs and repeat.

Check out www.bestlife.com to view video demonstrations for each exercise.

SAFE, EFFECTIVE STRETCHING

Your flexibility—the range of motion available in a joint, such as the shoulder, or a series of joints, such as the spine—is determined partly by genetics. But stretching regularly can help improve your flexibility. On the flip side, you can lose flexibility if you don't make stretching a habit. What does flexibility do for you? Some of the benefits:

- Reduces lower back pain

- Reduces cramping in the calves and quadriceps (upper leg muscles)

- Improves posture; helps prevent rounded shoulders

- Helps muscles relax, which can improve performance in exercise or any sporting activity, as well as everyday activities such as laundry, picking things up off the floor, or making the bed

- Speeds recovery from injury or training

- May reduce the chance of suffering an injury

- Improves mood and increases alertness

As stretching has become part of the exercise norm, many questions have come up about how and when to do it. Let's address them one by one.

Never stretch a cold muscle. At rest, there is less blood flow to the muscles and tendons, making them stiffer. Think of your muscles as rubber bands or bubble gum: If you stretch either of these when they are cold, they might snap. Stretch them when they're warm, however, and they will stretch more easily. Same for muscles.

Stretch after—not before—a cardio workout or light warm-up. Again, you don't want to stretch a cold muscle, and you'll get the most benefit from stretching when exercise has increased the blood flow to your muscles.

Don't bounce. Repeatedly moving up and down in a stretch can actually cause a tiny amount of damage (called microtrauma) in the muscle. Once damaged, the muscle works diligently to repair itself, which can create scar tissue. Scar tissue then makes the muscle less pliable, causing a decrease in flexibility. Stretch to the point where you feel a mild tug but no pain, and hold it there.

Hold stretches for 15 to 30 seconds. The greatest change in flexibility has been shown to happen in the first 15 seconds, and no significant improvement occurs after 30 seconds. Release, then repeat the stretch at least two times but no more than four times. More than that has not been shown to confer any significant improvement.

Stretch all major muscles. While some stretches feel better than others, it's important to give equal time to all your muscle groups to keep the body in balance. This includes the hamstrings, calves, lower back, shoulders, middle and upper back, and chest.

Stretch for yourself. Don't try to mimic what someone else is doing. Flexibility is very individualized, so listen to your body and challenge yourself within your own limits.

Don't follow the "no pain, no gain" adage. Again, when you're stretching, you should go until you feel tightness but not pain. If you feel pain, back off a bit. Back off, too, if you feel sore the day after stretching—you're probably overdoing it.

Consider taking a yoga or Pilates class. Both of these practices can help improve overall flexibility and strength.

The Plan, Part 2: Cardio

These days, aerobic exercise is more often called cardio, a nod to the fact that it accelerates your heart rate and improves your cardiovascular system. Cardio exercise not only gets your heart working harder, it also pushes your lungs to take in more air. By doing so, it ensures that your body can pump enough nutrient- and oxygen-laden blood to your working muscles to keep them going. It's like filling the gas tank of a car for a road trip. This process (and I'm just giving you a quick description of a complicated system) requires a fair amount of energy, which is why cardio exercise is the type of activity that burns the most calories. And, as you probably know, the harder and faster you do a cardio workout, the more calories you burn.

The number of different cardio workouts available to you is endless. Just to name a few: brisk walking, jogging or running (treadmill or outdoors), hiking, swimming, road cycling, mountain biking, spinning, stationary cycling, rowing machine, running or walking stairs, stair-stepping machine, elliptical trainer, inline skating, jumping rope, hip-hop aerobic dance, jazz dance. They're all good—although workouts that cause you to support all or most of your body weight with your own muscles (such as walking, running, aerobic dance, and stair climbing) challenge your body the most and ultimately help you burn the most calories. But that doesn't matter if you're not going to do the workout, so choose an activity that you like (or like enough to do regularly), is accessible (don't choose cycling if the road near your house is covered with snow four months out of the year), and fits your schedule and current fitness level.

Some people cannot (or will not) exercise in any structured fashion. That doesn't mean you can't exercise. Get yourself a pedometer and count the steps you take during the day as you go about your regular routine, taking care to walk as much as possible by, say, parking far from your destination, taking the stairs instead of elevators and escalators, and doing your errands on foot. Your ultimate goal should be to work up to eighteen thousand steps a day. To get that amount under your belt, you will probably have to adopt a slightly more structured approach and actually go for walks rather than just depend on getting the steps in through your regular routine. Still, all those everyday steps will add up and shorten the distance of your more formal walks.

If you're just beginning to exercise, check with your doctor beforehand. Then if she gives the okay, three days per week is a good starting point. But as you progress, and your fitness improves, add extra days. Working out more frequently not only increases the benefits, it also teaches you to make fitness a regular part of your routine, and that will help you maintain consistency. Be sure to exercise for at least thirty minutes. When you do so, you not only burn an ample number of calories but you also trigger more of the enzyme changes that boost your metabolism so that you burn more calories *after* exercises, too. Exercising for thirty minutes or more will also raise your core temperature, and that will most likely dull your appetite, making it easier to cut calories. If thirty minutes feels like an eternity, begin with fifteen minutes of exercise and then add two to three minutes to each successive workout. Within a few weeks, you'll be up to thirty minutes. From there, concentrate on working up to the goals I gave you on pages 156–157. I'll repeat them in brief here:

If you are aiming for weight loss or weight maintenance, 6 hours of moderately high-intensity exercise per week is the gold standard. For health benefits alone, 2½ hours of moderate-intensity cardio per week or 75 minutes of moderately high intensity per week is adequate.

Go back to chapter 4 to read about the details and some variations that might suit you.

The Plan, Part 3: Strength Training

Incorporating strength training into your routine will help you increase your lean muscle mass, a change that will benefit you in many ways. Muscle tissue requires more calories to maintain than fat. Therefore, with increased muscle mass, your body will burn a greater number of calories as part of its daily upkeep—even when you're sleeping or sitting around doing nothing. Another benefit of increasing muscle is that it helps prevent the natural loss of muscle tissue that occurs naturally with aging. Strength training also reinforces the skeleton, helping to stem bone loss and reducing your risk for osteoporosis. Last but not least, strength training gives your muscles the ability to perform quickly and efficiently.

There are hundreds of different strength-training exercises, but don't let the abundance of options confuse you. If you're really interested in strength training, I encourage you to learn more about the various exercises. However, there are eight simple moves (I call them the basic eight) that provide a great fundamental workout. Whether you've never lifted weights before or are an experienced exerciser who has never found the right strength-training regimen, you'll find the basic eight straightforward and not at all intimidating.

It takes surprisingly little time to do these exercises: just about twenty minutes. All you need are a few dumbbells; or, if you have access to weight machines at the gym, all these moves (except for squats) have a machine alternative. Choose the size of your dumbbells (or adjustment on the weight machines) according to how many repetitions you can do. The weights must be heavy enough to fatigue your muscles after eight to ten reps.

Begin with one or two sets per exercise, eight to ten repetitions per set three times a week. (Take no more than 15 to 30 seconds between sets.) You may find that you can't finish the eight reps in the second set, but that's okay; it's evidence that you're working hard enough in the first set. As your strength improves, you'll eventually be able to complete both sets. After about four weeks, reassess. If you're making all your sets easily, add another set. Also check your weights. Are they heavy enough? If not, move up to the next dumbbell weight or adjust the weight machines. Keep reassessing every four to six weeks, and when you're ready for a new challenge, add another day. Your ultimate goal: three sets of each exercise doing eight to ten reps every other day.

The Basic Eight

SQUAT

Works upper legs (quadriceps, hamstrings)

Stand with feet slightly wider than shoulder width apart, your back straight, head up, and toes and knees pointed slightly out. There should be a slight bend in your knees. Hold a dumbbell in each hand, your arms at your sides and palms facing inward. Contract your abdominal muscles. Bend your knees and gradually lower your body (as if you were going to sit in a chair) until your thighs are almost parallel with the floor; never let them go past parallel with the floor. Control your movements throughout the exercise, inhaling on the way down, exhaling on your way up. Pause for a second, then push up from your heels and gradually return to starting position.

LUNGE

Works upper and lower legs (quadriceps, hamstrings, gastrocnemius)

Stand with your feet shoulder width apart, your back straight, head up, and knees slightly bent. Hold a dumbbell in each hand, your arms at your sides and palms facing inward. Contract your abdominal muscles. Step forward with your right foot and bend both knees so that your front thigh becomes parallel to the floor. Your front knee should be directly above your ankle, never beyond it. Pause for a second and return to the starting position by pushing off from your front foot. Control your movement throughout the exercise, inhaling as you step forward, exhaling on the return. Repeat. Switch sides.

BUTTERFLY

Works upper back muscles (trapezius, latissimus dorsi)

Sit in a chair with your feet flat on floor. Keep your back flat against the back of the chair, with little or no arch. Hold a dumbbell in each hand, slightly above shoulder level and with palms facing each other, elbows bent, forearms parallel to each other in front of chest. Keep forearms about 4 or 5 inches apart and elbows close to your body. Contract your abs and the muscles of your upper back while you rotate your shoulders back in a semicircle, bringing elbows out to side. Keep both dumbbells above shoulder height throughout the exercise, pause for a second, and gradually return to starting position. Control your movements throughout the exercise, exhaling while rotating the dumbbells out and inhaling on the return.

DUMBBELL FLY

Works chest muscles (pectorals)

Lie on your back on a bench with your knees bent and your feet flat on the floor. Keep your back flat against the bench, with little or no arch and your arms fully extended but not hyperextended above your chest. Hold a dumbbell in each hand, palms facing inward. Contract your abdominal muscles. Gradually lower dumbbells out to the side, keeping elbows slightly bent throughout the exercise. Continue until upper arms are parallel with floor. Pause for a second, then gradually return to starting position. Control movements throughout the exercise, exhaling while lowering the dumbbells and inhaling on the return.

BICEPS CURL
Works upper arms (biceps)

Stand with your feet slightly apart and knees slightly bent. Hold a dumbbell in each hand, using an underhand grip, your arms at your sides and your palms facing inward. Contract abdominals. Curl the dumbbells up to your shoulder while twisting your palms so that they are facing you at the top of the move. Pause for a second and then gradually lower dumbbells to starting position. Control movements throughout the exercise, exhaling while lifting the dumbbells up and inhaling on the return.

TRICEPS EXTENSION
Works backs of the arms (triceps)

Stand with your feet slightly apart and your knees slightly bent, with your arms fully extended but not hyperextended above your head. Hold one dumbbell, using an interlocking grip. Contract your abdominal muscles. Gradually lower the dumbbell back behind your head and neck while keeping elbows in place above your head. Continue until forearms are parallel to floor, pause for a second, then gradually raise dumbbell to starting position. Control movements throughout the exercise, inhaling while lowering the dumbbell and exhaling while raising it back up.

CHEST PRESS
Works chest and backs of upper arms (pectorals, triceps)

Lie on your back on a bench with your knees bent and your feet on the floor.

Keep your back flat against the bench, with little or no arch. Hold a dumbbell in each hand slightly above chest level, with your palms facing forward. Contract your abdominal muscles. Gradually raise the dumbbells until your arms are fully extended above your chest. Do not hyperextend your elbows. Pause for a second, then gradually return dumbbells to starting position. Control your movements throughout the exercise, exhaling while raising the dumbbells and inhaling on the return.

SHOULDER PRESS
Works shoulder muscles (deltoids)

Sit upright on a chair or slightly slanted if using an incline bench, with your back supported and your feet flat on the floor. Keep your back flat against the back of the chair, with little or no arch. Hold a dumbbell in each hand slightly above shoulder level and with your palms facing forward, elbows out to the side. Contract your abdominals. Keeping palms facing forward, raise the dumbbells up and inward until the inside ends of dumbbells are nearly touching each other and are directly overhead. Do not hyperextend your elbows. Pause for a second, then gradually lower the dumbbells to starting position. Control your movements throughout the exercise, exhaling while raising the dumbbells and inhaling on the return.

Check out www.bestlife.com to view video demonstrations for each exercise.

Pulling It All Together: Twelve-Week Fitness Plan

How you approach this twelve-week plan depends on your present level of fitness. If you're starting at zero—meaning that you haven't exercised for months or years, or maybe have never done any kind of formal exercise at all—I suggest that you follow the "Pre-plan" Plan that starts on page 271. That will help get you up to speed so that you can comfortably start the twelve-week regimen at the beginning level without fear of injury or overexertion. No matter what level you are at now, rest assured that the Twelve-Week Fitness Plan allows for a gradual increase in duration, frequency, and intensity.

To begin, determine your current activity level in the box below, then use that as your starting point. (Again, get your doctor's okay before beginning.) While the program runs twelve weeks, you can repeat it all year long, either staying at the level that you initially worked up to or continuing to move up. For instance, if you're currently at level 1 but eventually want to reach level 3, then start week 1 at level 1. As you can see, you'll switch to level 2 by the fifth week, finishing off the twelve weeks at level 2. Ready for level 3? Then go ahead and restart the twelve-week cycle at level 3 this time. If you need a few more weeks at level 2, start the cycle at level 2 again and progress when you feel ready.

Note: If you are at level 4, assume that week 5 is your starting point. Then when you get to what is everyone else's week 12 (but your week 8), repeat it for another four weeks. While we show you how to make the transition from levels 4 to 5, this program really isn't for level 5 exercisers. If you are at level 5, think about new ways that you can challenge yourself, such as training for a competition like a 10K race, mixing in another activity to your routine, or joining an athletic workout group.

FIND YOUR ACTIVITY LEVEL

Read through the six levels below to determine your activity level.

You're at activity level 0 if: You don't do any activity except what you need to get you through your day. You don't do any formal exercise and avoid any extra movement by doing things like parking close to your destination and always taking the elevator instead of the stairs.

YOUR CURRENT EXERCISE TOTALS
Aerobic exercise: none

or
Steps per day: 3,499 or less
Strength training: none

You're at activity level 1 if: You have an active job, like waitressing or teaching, but you don't do any formal exercise. Or maybe you try to work off a few calories by walking to the store rather than driving, going down the hall to talk to colleagues instead of calling or emailing, or riding bikes with your kids.

YOUR CURRENT EXERCISE TOTALS

Aerobic exercise: up to 90 minutes per week; if you haven't done aerobic exercise in a while, keep the intensity moderate.
or
Steps per day: approximately 3,500 to 5,999
Strength training: none

You're at activity level 2 if: You have a consistent, structured exercise routine, although it's very moderate. You get in about three thirty-minute sessions a week.

YOUR CURRENT EXERCISE TOTALS

Aerobic exercise: five times a week, at least 90 to 150 minutes per week
or
Steps per day: approximately 6,000 to 9,999
Strength training: at least three times a week, a minimum of eight exercises

You're at activity level 3 if: You work out five or six days a week, include cardiovascular exercise into your routine, and strength train two days a week.

YOUR CURRENT EXERCISE TOTALS

Aerobic exercise: five times a week, 150 to 250 minutes per week
or
Steps per day: approximately 10,000 to 13,999
Strength training: at least two times a week, a minimum of six exercises

You're at activity level 4 if: You work out almost every day. Along with strength training three days a week, you cross train aerobically, maybe alternating among jogging, going to spin class, and swimming.

YOUR CURRENT EXERCISE TOTALS

Aerobic exercise: five times a week, at least 250 to 360 minutes per week
or
Steps per day: approximately 14,000 to 17,999
Strength training: at least three times a week, a minimum of eight exercises

You're at activity level 5 if: Exercising is your way of life. You rarely miss a day of working out, do everything level 4 does and even more, maybe by doing ten different strength-training exercises per session and/or training for running, cycling, or swimming competitions.

YOUR CURRENT EXERCISE TOTALS

Aerobic exercise: seven times a week, 360 minutes or more per week
or
Steps per day: approximately 18,000 or above
Strength training: at least three times a week, a minimum of ten exercises

THE "PRE-PLAN" PLAN

WEEK 1 TO 4	LEVEL 0
FUNCTIONAL FITNESS	**WALKING**
Do all the functional fitness stretches and strengtheners, 7 days a week	Walk at a pace of 7 on the Perceived Exertion Scale, 10 to 15 minutes, 3 days per week

TWELVE-WEEK FITNESS PLAN

WEEKS 1 TO 2

CARDIO

Beginner (Level 1)	Intermediate (Level 2)	Advanced (Level 3)
20 minutes (or as much as you can do), at least 3 days per week	40 minutes, 3 days per week	45 minutes, 5 days per week

STRENGTH TRAINING

Beginner (None)	Intermediate (None)	Advanced (Level 3)
		6 to 8 strength-training moves, 1 to 2 sets of 8 to 10 repetitions, 2 days per week

FUNCTIONAL FITNESS

Everyone: Do all the stretches and strengtheners, 7 days a week

WEEKS 3 TO 4

CARDIO

Beginner (Level 1)	Intermediate (Level 2)	Advanced (Level 3)
Add 5 more minutes of cardio to each workout for a total of 25 minutes, at least 3 days per week	Add 5 more minutes of cardio to each workout for a total of 45 minutes, 3 days per week	Add 5 more minutes of cardio to each workout for a total of 50 minutes, 5 days per week

STRENGTH TRAINING

Beginner (None)	Intermediate (None)	Advanced
		Repeat the routine from weeks 1 and 2

FUNCTIONAL FITNESS

Everyone: Do all the stretches and strengtheners, 7 days a week

Congratulations, you are moving up to the next level! If moving up is too challenging, stay at your current level until you feel comfortable moving up. You'll know you're ready when your workout feels challenging but is no longer difficult.

WEEKS 5 TO 6

CARDIO

Beginner (Level 2)	Intermediate (Level 3)	Advanced (Level 4)
Add 5 more minutes of cardio to each workout for a total of 30 minutes, 3 days per week	Do only 30 minutes of cardio *but* add 2 days for a total of 5 days per week	Add 5 more minutes of cardio to each workout for a total of 55 minutes, 5 days per week

STRENGTH TRAINING

Beginner (None)	Intermediate (Level 3)	Advanced (Level 4)
	6 strength-training moves; 1 to 2 sets of 8 to 10 repetitions, 2 days per week	8 strength-training moves; 3 sets of 8 to 10 repetitions, 3 days per week

FUNCTIONAL FITNESS

Everyone

Do all the stretches and strengtheners, 7 days a week

WEEKS 7 TO 8

CARDIO

Beginner (Level 2)	Intermediate (Level 3)	Advanced (Level 4)
Add 5 more minutes of cardio to each workout for a total of 35 minutes, 3 days per week	Add 5 more minutes of cardio to each workout for a total of 35 minutes, 5 days per week	Add 5 more minutes of cardio to each workout for a total of 60 minutes, 5 days per week

STRENGTH TRAINING

Beginner (None)	Intermediate (Level 3)	Advanced (Level 4)
	Repeat the routine from weeks 5 and 6	Repeat the routine from weeks 5 and 6

FUNCTIONAL FITNESS

Everyone

Do all the stretches and strengtheners, 7 days a week

WEEKS 9 TO 10

CARDIO

Beginner (Level 2)	Intermediate (Level 3)	Advanced (Level 4)
Add 5 more minutes of cardio to each workout for a total of 40 minutes, 3 days per week	Add 10 more minutes of cardio to each workout for a total of 45 minutes, 5 days per week	Add 5 more minutes of cardio to each workout for a total of 65 minutes, 5 days per week

STRENGTH TRAINING

Beginner (None)	Intermediate (Level 3)	Advanced (Level 4)
	6 to 8 strength-training moves; 3 sets of 8 to 10 repetitions, 2 days per week	Repeat the routine from weeks 5 and 6

FUNCTIONAL FITNESS

Everyone

Do all the stretches and strengtheners, 7 days a week

WEEKS 11 TO 12

CARDIO

Beginner (Level 2)

Add 10 more minutes of cardio to each workout for a total of 50 minutes, 3 days per week

Intermediate (Level 3)

Add 5 more minutes of cardio to each workout for a total of 50 minutes, 5 days per week

Advanced (Level 5)

(This is to demonstrate what it's like to reach level 5. If you're not prepared for the greater exercise commitment, then stay at level 4.) Add 10 more minutes of cardio to each workout for a total of 75 minutes, 5 days per week

STRENGTH TRAINING

Beginner (None)

Intermediate (Level 3)

6 to 8 strength-training moves; 3 sets of 8 to 10 repetitions, 3 days per week

Advanced (Level 5)

Repeat the routine from weeks 5 and 6

FUNCTIONAL FITNESS

Everyone

Do all the stretches and strengtheners, 7 days a week

Congratulations! You can now move up to the next activity level or stay right where you are until you are more comfortable. Remember to keep challenging yourself, but don't move up before you are ready. This isn't a rush to the finish line—this is a lifelong commitment to yourself.

Exercising with a Chronic Condition

The title above says it all: You *can* exercise with a chronic condition, whether it's heart disease, diabetes, or fibromyalgia. Starting on page 155 in chapter 4, I covered general exercise guidelines. Check in with your doctor to see if it's okay to follow those guidelines and the twelve-week plan. If not, work with your doctor to see if you're able to follow the condition-specific suggestions below.

ARTHRITIS (OSTEOARTHRITIS OR RHEUMATOID ARTHRITIS)

Your exercise Rx: Physical activity is especially effective in helping reduce the symptoms of rheumatoid arthritis. It can work almost like a drug, beating back inflammation and reducing pain and stiffness. If you have either type of arthritis, go for low-impact activities that won't further damage your joints. Low impact doesn't necessarily mean low intensity: Work up to moderate or high intensity unless your doctor recommends otherwise. (People with osteoarthritis have to be particularly careful and work within their abilities.) Some examples of low-impact workouts: swimming or other water exercises (warm water is probably best for you); riding a stationary bike (either upright or recumbent) or cycling outdoors on flat terrain; and walking. The elliptical trainer works well for a lot of people—just make sure that it doesn't cause any pain. Wear supportive athletic shoes that are very shock absorbent. Most people with arthritis can handle resistance training, and, in fact, it will strengthen the muscles around your weakened joints and help you function better.

   Special concerns: If your ankles, knees, and/or hips have been damaged, even walking might be too much of a strain, so stick to the other suggested activities. As for strength training, keep weights light enough to allow you to easily do ten reps, and increase weights very slowly. The resistance should never become too challenging, or you could further damage your joints.

DIABETES

Your exercise Rx: Because 70 percent of deaths from type 2 diabetes are a result of secondary heart disease, your prescription is the same as anyone trying to prevent heart disease: regular moderate- to high-intensity aerobic workouts. If you can safely tolerate moderately high-intensity exercise (7 or 8 on the Perceived Exertion Scale, pages 158–160), then go for it, because it's best for lowering blood sugar. Both aerobic exercise and strength training improve insulin sensitivity, so incorporate both into your regimen. For more information on exercising with diabetes, see *The Best Life Guide to Managing Diabetes and Pre-Diabetes* or go to www.thebestlife.com/diabetes.

Special concerns: If you also have heart disease, check out recommendations for exercising with that condition elsewhere in this section. Before, during, and after exercise, monitor your blood sugar: If your blood sugar is below 100 before working out, have a snack that contains 15 grams of carbohydrate, such as 4 ounces of fruit juice. Retest in fifteen minutes. Start exercising when your sugar exceeds 100 and test throughout. (If sugar drops, have another 15-gram carbohydrate snack.) If your blood sugar is higher than 300 before exercise, wait until it drops below that number before starting your workout. The same thing goes for ketones: If you test high, wait until they drop. If you're taking insulin or other drugs that cause you to make more insulin (such as sulfonylureas and meglitinides), you may be particularly prone to a hypoglycemic (low blood sugar) reaction to exercise. In that case, consult your doctor about reducing your dose of medication on exercise days. If you have diabetic neuropathy in the feet—a common complication of diabetes—avoid high-impact activities like jogging and instead opt for cycling, swimming, walking, and other lower-impact exercises.

FIBROMYALGIA

Your exercise Rx: Because fibromyalgia symptoms include muscle pain and tender points on areas of the body, it's important to keep impact at a minimum. Walking, elliptical exercise, cycling, tai chi, dance, water exercises in warm water, and other low-impact aerobic activities done at moderate intensity (or low intensity if necessary) are usually best. Strength training helps combat muscle weakness associated with the condition; build up gradually, as tolerated. On those days when fatigue makes it hard to get out the door (or even out of bed), remember that exercise can be invigorating. It also has benefits that may help relieve your condition, such as reducing inflammation and enhancing sleep.

Special concerns: High-impact activities may cause pain, and working out at high intensity may leave you more exhausted than energized.

HEART DISEASE (CORONARY ARTERY DISEASE)

Your exercise Rx: With your doctor's blessing, you can do most types of aerobic exercise at moderate intensity. Bump up the intensity only with your doctor's sign-off and work with him or her on how to progress. You should be doing the functional fitness exercises on pages 257 to 260 and, again with the doc's permission, strength training.

Special concerns: While the benefits of exercise outweigh the small risk that it can trigger a heart attack, you still need to approach it cautiously. Before starting a new exercise regimen or before raising the intensity level of activities you're already doing, consult with your doctor. If you've been sedentary, work up slowly to a higher intensity. According to the American Heart Association, everyone with heart disease should warm up for five minutes before exercising and cool down for five minutes at the end. Your doctor may have set a maximum heart rate limit during workouts, especially if you've had a heart attack or chest pain (angina). Use a heart rate monitor to stay within that limit. If nitroglycerine (it opens up blood vessels, allowing more blood to flow to organs, and can reduce chest pain) was prescribed, make sure to have it handy while exercising.

Strength training raises blood pressure, so you might have to limit the amount of weights and reps you do—again, discuss this with your physician. If you have certain conditions, such as uncontrolled hypertension or arrhythmias (abnormal cardiac rhythms, such as skipping a beat), your doctor may nix strength training altogether. But if you get the medical okay, start with a lower resistance on machines or free weights. "Low" means that you can perform ten reps relatively easily.

LOW BACK PAIN

Your exercise Rx: As long as it doesn't hurt your back, do low-impact aerobic exercise (such as walking, cycling, swimming, using the elliptical machine), strength training, and functional exercises. Functional exercises are particularly important for preventing reinjury; for instance, the crunches and arm and leg raises described on pages 257 to 259 strengthen your back muscles, and stretching improves flexibility.

Special concerns: If you feel any back pain while doing any sort of exercise, stop immediately. While yoga, Pilates, and tai chi can strengthen your back and improve flexibility, they can also hurt your back if you push yourself beyond comfortable limits. Don't get competitive in these classes!

For the first two weeks after back pain hits, stick to low-impact aerobics (and check with your doctor, who may also recommend low-intensity exercise). Also, for at least two weeks, lay off crunches or any other functional fitness moves involving the trunk. Resume when the pain subsides.

OSTEOPOROSIS

Your exercise Rx: Exercise, particularly weight-bearing exercise, in combination with a class of drugs called bisphosphonates, can actually strengthen and thicken your bones. So do the full range of recommended exercises (aerobic, strength training, and functional), keeping in mind the caveats below.

Special concerns: Although it's the impact of an exercise—the stress you put on your muscles and joints as your feet hit the ground—that stimulates bone growth, you have to be careful not to fracture fragile bones with too much impact. So unless your doctors says otherwise, do low-impact activities, such as walking, the exercise bike, or outdoor cycling on flat terrain. If your osteoporosis is severe, you may have to stick to swimming, which is considered "no impact."

Strength training also builds bone, especially when you use relatively heavier weights and fewer reps. Be careful when doing any exercises that involve bending forward and twisting the spine; either skip them or modify them so that you don't bend and twist as far. With any type of exercise, reduce your risk for falling by avoiding unstable surfaces, keeping any obstacles out of the way, and, if necessary, using a chair or the wall for balance and support.

INDEX

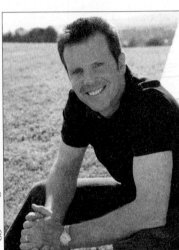

Reggie Casagrande

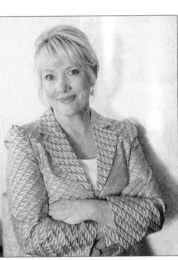

Michael Molinoff

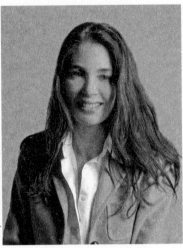

Abby Greenawalt

About the Authors

Bob Greene is an exercise physiologist and certified personal trainer specializing in fitness, metabolism, and weight loss. He has been a guest on *The Oprah Winfrey Show.* He is also a contributing writer and editor for *O: The Oprah Magazine* and writes articles on health and fitness for Oprah.com. Bob is the bestselling author of *The Best Life Guide to Managing Diabetes and Pre-Diabetes, The Best Life Diet Cookbook, The Best Life Diet,* and *Get with the Program!,* among other books. Visit his website at www.thebestlife.com.

Ann Kearney-Cooke, PhD, is the director of the Cincinnati Psychotherapy Institute. She has been named a distinguished scholar for the Partnership for Women's Health at Columbia University in New York, where she developed the curriculum for the Helping Girls Become Strong Women Project. She has lectured at more than 150 conferences and written on body image, self-esteem, and the treatment of eating disorders. Ann is the psychological expert for the Weight Loss Diary column in *Shape* magazine, and her work has been featured on shows such as NBC's *Today,* CBS's *The Morning Show,* and *The Oprah Winfrey Show.*

Janis Jibrin, MS, RD, is the lead nutritionist for www.thebestlife.com, Bob Greene's weight loss and fitness website. A contributing editor for *Self* magazine, she is the author of *The Supermarket Diet* and other weight-loss books and freelances for national magazines. She was a coauthor of *The Best Life Guide to Managing Diabetes and Pre-Diabetes.* In her private practice, she specializes in weight loss and eating disorders.